The Way of Thinking in Chinese Medicine

Culture and Knowledge
Edited by Friedrich G. Wallner

Vol. 13

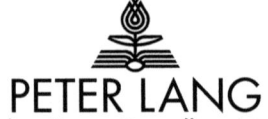

PETER LANG
Frankfurt am Main · Berlin · Bern · Bruxelles · New York · Oxford · Wien

Friedrich G. Wallner
Fengli Lan
Martin J. Jandl
(eds.)

The Way of Thinking in Chinese Medicine

Theory, Methodology and Structure
of Chinese Medicine

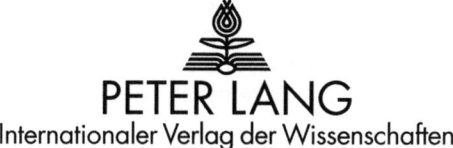

PETER LANG
Internationaler Verlag der Wissenschaften

Bibliographic Information published by the Deutsche Nationalbibliothek
The Deutsche Nationalbibliothek lists this publication in the Deutsche Nationalbibliografie; detailed bibliographic data is available in the internet at http://dnb.d-nb.de.

Cover illustration:
"Nike von Samothraki"
Courtesy of Kovac-Verlag.

Printed with financial support of the Federal Ministry of Science and Research in Vienna.

ISSN 1613-902X
ISBN 978-3-631-61196-8
© Peter Lang GmbH
Internationaler Verlag der Wissenschaften
Frankfurt am Main 2010
All rights reserved.

All parts of this publication are protected by copyright. Any utilisation outside the strict limits of the copyright law, without the permission of the publisher, is forbidden and liable to prosecution. This applies in particular to reproductions, translations, microfilming, and storage and processing in electronic retrieval systems.

www.peterlang.de

Table of Contents

Vincent Shen
Dao, Qi, and Body/Mind-Huanglao Daoist Methodology of Nurturing Life 7

Lan Fengli
Globalization of TCM: Cultural Differences between TCM and Western Medicine 24

Gertrude Kubiena
Applied Methodologies for Teaching, Learning, Spreading and Survival of TCM 45

Lan Fengli
Metaphor, *Qu Xiang Bi Lei* and Chinese Medicine 63

Pan Guijuan
Discussion of the Basic Categories in the TCM Theoretical System 89

Ma Xiaotong
TCM Essential Conception and Methods of the Theory 95

Fritz G. Wallner & Lan Fengli
Ontological Ambiguity and Methodological Circularity: *QU-XIANG BI-LEI* 103

Sophie Chung
Structural Paralellisms in Psychoanalysis and Traditional Chinese Medicine and Their Struggle for Scientific Acknowledgement in the Western World 118

Vincent Shen

Dao, Qi, and Body/Mind-Huanglao Daoist Methodology of Nurturing Life

Introduction

This paper will mainly explore the theory and practice of nurturing life (養生 *yangsheng*) and cultivating mind (*xiuxin* 修心) in the Chapter *Neiye* 內業 (Inner Working) of the *Guanzi* 管子, one of the founding texts of Huanglao Daoism on which most of the philosophy of Chinese medicine is based. Although nurturing life and curing of disease are like the two wheels of the same vehicle of Chinese medicine, the priority should be given always to the nurturing of life, which means not only the maintaining of life functions but also the growing of life itself, if well done there would be much less or even no disease to be cured. Since body and mind are so closely related to each other, the nurturing of life is also closely related to the cultivation of mind. Here we are dealing with a theory of preventive medicine rather than that of curative medicine.

In the following, I'll present a concept of "methodology" different from that in the western context of "logic, methodology and philosophy of science", which inevitably involved western philosophical concepts and theories of science and methodology that would trap Traditional Chinese Medicine (TCM) in their methodological considerations without allowing the later to develop its own methodology. Instead, I'll discuss "methodology" as in its deeper relation with the movement of reality and human practice: this means I'll be dealing with methodology as dynamic ontology and practical methodology in the line of thought of TCM, all in using some Huanglao Daoist texts to illustrate this point. In this context, I'll discuss the nurturing of life and its necessary connection to the cultivation of mind, rather than the curing of diseases.

Indeed, when we read Huanglao texts such as the Inner Working, methodology was seen there as unified with ontology. In it, the Dao was considered both as the Ultimate Reality and as the Way, in reference to which the methodology of nurturing life (*yang sheng* 養生) and cultivating mind/heart (*xiu xin* 修心) should be considered. Somehow like Hegel who took Spirit (*Geist*) as the True Reality and, based on it, all methodology should be dealing with the methods and steps by which the Spirit goes out of its own familiarity in order to return and eventually to fulfill itself. Similarly, for the Huanglao Daoists, the Dao is the Ultimate Reality, that which gives life to all things, and accordingly, the methodology of keeping life in good condition should take into account the way by which the Dao gives life and keeps the life of myriad things. Also, in order to render the concept of the Dao pragmatic, in its relevance to the functioning of the universe, the governing of the State and the conservation of life, the concept of *jing qi* 精氣 (Subtle Vital Energy), was proposed as that by which the Dao gives life to myriad things in the universe, that which conserves life and allows life to growth as it should be.

Here we need a short historical note on the Huanglao Daoism. For me, there were three phases in the development of Classical Daoism:
- 1st Phase: Laozi 老子 (6th Century BCE)
- 2nd Phase: Zhuangzi 莊子 (399?-295?BCE)
- 3rd Phase: Huanglao 黃老 Daoism (4th - 2nd Century BCE)

Huanglao Daoism emerged at the late middle Warring State when time and society demanded more active and pragmatic contribution from the Daoists. Huanglao Daoism emerged in a time of transition from the social-political disorder of late Warring States to the reestablishment of order in Han Dynasty. Also, Huanglao Daoism served as the transition from Philosophical Daoism to Religious Daoism, with their method and art of conserving life, searching for longevity and cultivation of authentic person, and eventually for the ideal of immortality, so attractive not only to common people but especially to those in power of the time. The application of the Daoist ideas of laws of nature (*tiandao* 天道 or *tiandi zhi dao* 天地之道) to the governance of the state and the methods of nurturing life (*yangsheng*) and cultivation of mind/heart (*xiu xin*) must have constituted a major part of their advices to the kings and political leaders of the time. Now their discourses are available for us, not only as historical documents, but also as useful advices today for a holistic vision of preventive medicine and self-cultivation.

Historically, we can divide Huanglao Daoism into two different branches. The first started earlier, in the 4th Century BC, in the state of

Chu, which was said to be the native country of Loazi. The representative texts of this south branch of Huanglao Daoism was the *Huanglao Silk Texts*, or, according to some scholars, the *Four Classics of Yellow Emperor (Huangdi Sijing* 黃帝四經)[1]. The other branch emerged in connection with Jixia Academy of the state of Qi in the north, with the Daoist members of that Academy. This second branch could have received influence from Huanglao Daoism of the south and developed their ideas in the particular context of Jixia Academy. The most representative works of this branch of Huanglao Daoism were the *"Four Daoist Chapters of the Guanzi"* (管子四篇), though some Daoist ideas could still be found in some other chapters of that book as product of Qi scholars.[2]

The *Guangzi* could be seen as composed by the local scholars of Qi state, who, in facing the competition of different schools of thought in the Jixia Academy, referred themselves to Guang Zhong (d. 645BC), the most famous legalist master thinker and prime minister of Qi State, to feature the contribution of local thinkers at a time when "hundred schools compete to voice themselves", all in absorbing and synthesizing other schools of thought such as Daoism, Confucianism and Mohism. Among the now existing 76 chapters of the *Guangzi*, the Jixia Huanglao Daoist Writings could be found basically in the four chapters entitled *Technique of Heart* (Xinshu 心術) I and II, *Inner Working* (Neiye 內業) and Cleaning the Heart (Baixin 白心). In the Chapter *Inner Working*, the influence of Confucianism, especially the idealist Confucianism of Mencius is obvious from its use of the concept of *xin* (mind).

---

[1] See, *Huangdi sijing jinzhujinyi*(Commentary and translation of *Four Classics of Yellow Emperor* in modern Chinese), Commentary and translation by Guying Chen, Taipei: Commercial Press, 1995. English translations in this paper are mine. The Chinese texts hereafter abbreviated as *Four Classics*.

[2] The Chinese text I use refers to the *Guanzi Jiaozheng*(Guanzi Proofread and Corrected), Commented by Yin Zhizhang, proofread and corrected by Dai Wang, reprint, Taipei: World Bookstore, 1981. (Hereafter referred to as the *Guanzi*). Usually the English translations in this paper are mine. However, there is an English translation: *Guanzi A Study and translation* by W. Allyn Rickett, revised edition, 2 volumes, Boston: Cheng and Tsui Company, 2001. From time to time, my translation has consulted Rickett's in correcting it by my own reading of the Chinese texts.

Dao and Qi in the Huang Lao Silk Texts

A general characteristic of the Huanglao texts was that, though they still took Dao as the Ultimate Reality, they preferred to use the concept of *qi* when discussing the problems related to the origin and function of the universe. For example, in the representative text of the Southern Huanglao Daoists, the *Huanglao Silk Texts* did not indulge themselves in discussing the Dao in itself. They emphasized rather the Dao as origin of all things and all activities in the world. Their description of this Original state of the universe could be read as a description of *qi*, such as:

"*In the beginning when nothing exists, the cosmos seems to exist in a state of undifferentiated sameness. There is nothing else in the void but the One. It was in a undifferentiated chaos without yet light and darkness, it was divinely marvelous and fulfilled everywhere, subtle, still and devoid of brightness. Therefore nothing seems to derive from it and nothing seems yet to depend on it. Therefore it is without any determinate form, indifferently same and without name. The Heaven can not cover it, the earth cannot support it, that which makes the small small, the big big. It is full in the four seas, and contains them from outside. It will not get rotted in its begotten ying, and not burnt in the yang. Its measure is unchangeable for everything and let all animals, big or small live in their own way. It let the bird fly, the fish swim, the beast run. It gives birth to myriad of things and let hundred events accomplish themselves.*" [1]

This text conceived the One, somehow like the One Qi of the *Zhuangzi*, as an undifferentiated and formless whole, filling up everywhere, giving birth and measure to all things. These were ostensive attributes of the One, therefore different from Laozi for whom Dao gave birth to the One, but itself was not the One, also all the attributes Laozi gave reluctantly to the Dao were but figurative attributes, not ostensive attributes. The reason of this was that *Huanglao Silk Texts* conceived the Dao as the One Qi, which was undifferentialted and fulfilled everywhere, and was not decreased or increased by the birth or death of all things.

"*Heaven and Earth, yin and yang, four seasons, sun and moon, stars and cloudy sky, all kind of animals and plants, all draw their life from it,*

---

[1] *Four Classics*, p.470

though it is not decreased thereby; all return to it after their death, yet it is not increase thereby."[1]

When the One self-differentiates itself into myriad things, it created oppositions such as bright and dark, ying and yang, and served as their unity. In the chapter *Guang* 觀 of the *Shidajing* 十大經, it was said,
"The Dao is without brightness and darkness, without yin and yang, when yin and yang are not yet determined, we could not even call it by name. And now, it begins to differentiate into two, separate into yin and yang, and divide into four seasons."[2]

This was quite different from the *Laozi* in which the Dao gave birth to myriad things, not by immediately self-differentiating into myriad things in oppositional states, but through the mediation of non-being and being, the two ontological moment of Dao's self-manifestation, before there emerged myriad things in opposition both structurally and dynamically. In some sense, the cosmology of *Huanglao Silk Texts* lacked the ontological depth of Laozi while concretizing it through its interpretation of the Dao as the One Qi. Also the *Huanglao Silk Texts* emphasized the anthropological aspect of the One in which the One becomes the origin and foundation of all human spirit and wisdom,

"The Dao is the origin of spiritual enlightenment. The spiritual enlightenment is that which, even when situated within the measure, still has vision beyond all measure.... When still, they are unchangeable; when acting, they are imperishable, that is why we call it the divine (spirit). The spiritual wisdom is the insight into the paradigm of all human knowledge."[3]

In short, *Huanglao Silk Texts* tended to interpret the Dao as One Qi and to emphasize the cosmological aspect of the Dao and to neglect its ontological aspect. The cosmological Dao became the foundation and justification of human beings' life praxis and the King's or political leader's self-cultivation and political action, not only as the ground of their wisdom, but also of their struggle for power and profit.

---

1 *Four Classics*, p.470
2 *Four Classics*, p.268
3 *Four Classics*, p.232

Onto-Methodology: Methodology as Ontology

As to the representative texts of the northern Huanglao Daoists, such as the *Neiye* (Inner Working), they, like Laozi, Zhuangzi and Daoists in general, took the Dao as the Ultimate Reality and the origin of all things, although they would put the emphasis on the Subtle Qi (精氣) by which the Dao gave life to myriad things. The Subtle Qi, though non-substantial and therefore inaudible, formless and non-active, was a reality much more tangible and therefore understandable than the Dao. In the *Neiye*, it said,

"*The Subtle is the essence of all things. It is with it that the Dao begins to give life. It gives life to the five grains down on the earth, and the stars up in the sky. When the Subtle Qi drifts between Heaven and earth, it is called the ghost and the divine. When stored in the bosom of a particular human being, this man would become a sage.*"[1]

"*What I mean by the Subtle is the Subtle of Qi, with which the Dao starts to give birth to life. Only when you have life that you can conduct meditation; only when you conduct meditation that you get [true knowledge]; Only when you have true knowledge that you know where to stop.*"[2]

We should say that, ontologically, the Dao preceded the Subtle Qi, which should be created by the Dao in order to give life to myriad things. This could be found in the recently discovered *Heng Xian* (The Constant Precedes…) in which we read,

"*The Constant preceded non-being and being. It was simple, quiet and void. To say it was simple, it was indeed the Great Simple; to say it was quiet, it was indeed the Great Quiet; to say it was void, it was indeed the Great Void. It was not satisfied with self-enclosure, therefore it rose to create the Space. Since there was Space, there was qi (the original stuff). Since there was qi, there were beings. Since there were beings, there was beginning. Since there was beginning, there was passing away.*"[3]

Here the term "Constant" (*Heng* 恆) was another name of Dao, whose existence, as was said in the text, preceded that of being and non-being, and, because of it's not satisfying with staying within itself, it went

---

1 The *Guanzi*, p.268
2 The *Guanzi*, p.270
3 See Hengxian, in *Shanghai Bowuguan Chang Zhanguo Chuzhushu* (Shanghai Collection of the Chu Bamboo Slips of Warring States) vol.III, Shanghai: Guji Press, 2003. pp.103, 288. My English translation.

out side of its self-enclosure and thereby creates Space and then Qi in the Space, and then myriad things. This is to say that Dao created myriad thing by not staying in its self-enclosure, on the contrary, it was by way of its original generosity that Dao went outside of itself to myriad things, an act that we may call "strangification", signifying the act of going outside of oneself to many others, to many strangers. We see this spirit of original generosity and metaphysical strangification very much emphasized by Laozi himself. The cosmic process itself was seen by him as the out come of such a generosity, as Laozi said, "[The Space] between Heaven and Earth, is it not like a bellows? Vacuous and yet inexhaustible, it moves and yet more comes out"[1], in which the phrase "the more comes out" discloses the original generosity of the Dao. And then, based on the original generosity of Dao and its metaphysical strangification to give birth to myriad things in the universe, the sage also led a life of generosity: "The sage does not accumulate for himself. The more he does for others, the richer is his life. The more he gives to others, the more he has within."[2]

In comparison, for Huanglao Daoism, due to its concern with the function and conservation of body/mind, the emphasis was not so much put on the ethical generosity but rather on the nurturing of life and the cultivation of mind/heart. This is to say that Huanglao Daoism served also the transition from Classical Daoist philosophy of transcendence to the later Daoists' philosophical and religious immanence.

Huanglao Daoism kept the same idea of Laozi that Dao Itself was the undifferentiated whole, and when It gave birth to myriad things in the process of differentiation and complexification, it got specific determination in everything and abode also in everything. The concrete determination of the Dao in each thing that served as the nature of each thing was called their "original power (*de* 德)". In the *Xinshu Shang* (Technique of Heart I), it was said,

"That which is void, non-being, formless is called the Dao; that which transforms and nourishes the life of all things is called the de" "The de is the dwelling of the Dao, by which things could be give birth...Dwelling is

---

1 Laozi, Chapter 5, in *Laozi Sizong* (Four versions of the *Laozi*) Taipei, Da An Publisher, 1999, p.4. My English translation.
2 Ibid., p.66. My English translation.

the de, therefore there is no distance between Dao and de, and those who propose discourse on them do not discriminate between them."[1]

We should say that *de* was the Dao inside each and every being. It was the original creative power of very being. It was only by way of preparing one's *de* that one could receive Dao and its life-giving Subtle Vital Energy (*jingqi*) in oneself. The *Neiye* we read, "Thus, this Subtle Vital Force is never to be stopped within one's self by physical strength. It may be brought to peaceful rest only by one's *de*."[2]

On the other hand, the Dao was also conceived as the Way, in this sense, it was the foundation of all "methodologies", or, as the *Neiye* put it, "the ordering of things into their achievement." We read, "The Way is that which fills the body/mind, although common men are unable to hold it in place. Going, it may not return; coming, it may not dwell. We cannot see its form, we cannot hear its sound, yet it is the order according to which one achieve one's life. That's why it's called the Dao."[3] In the following text, the onto-methodological meaning of the Dao was made even much clearer:

"*Dao is that which cannot be spoken by the mouth, cannot be seen by the eyes, cannot be heard by the ears. It is that by which one cultivates his mind (xiu xin) and rectifies one's body. When man loses it, men dies, when man gets it, he lives on; Events, when loses it, fails, succeeds when obtains it. The Dao is that by which myriads things live and achieves their purposes, that why it's named Dao.*"[4]

That the Way had its methodological meaning also based itself on the idea that it was the Dao that gave birth to Law/Method in the management of one's body and in the governance of the state, both founded on the Daoist concept of laws of nature, as Dao's manifestation in the regulation of the universes. In the beginning of the Chapter *Jingfa* of the *Huanglao Silk Texts*, it was said,

"*The Dao gives birth to Law/Method. Law/Method is that which refers to in judging loose and gain, as in the line of ink which discerns crook and right. He who governs by law, should promulgates law/method and do nothing against it.*"[5]

---

1 The *Guanzhi*, p.221
2 The *Guanzhi*, p.269
3 The *Guanzhi*, p.269
4 The *Guanzhi*, p.269
5 *Four Classics*, p.48

The Chinese term *fa* means both law and method. It is clear from this text that all laws/methods came from the Dao. In the *Huanglao Silk Texts*, the concept of law contained two layers of meaning. In its broad sense, it means the standard of measurement of all things and events. This is the Laws of nature conforming to which all things come into being. This aspect of law could also be named as li (理), the principle of all things. In this aspect, *Huanglao Silk Texts* followed Laozi's thought that, structurally speaking, all things were constituted of opposites; and dynamically speaking, when one state of affairs developed to its highest state, it went naturally to its opposite side. Also, in its strict sense, *fa* means also the positive laws or promulgated laws, which for the Huanglao Daoist should refer themselves to the Laws of Nature.

Within the conceptual framework of this onto/methodology, human beings was considered to have given birth by the harmonious cooperation of heaven and earth. It was heaven that gave birth to human essence or its subtle part, and it was the earth that gave birth to human body. We read, "It's ever so that in man's life, Heaven produces his subtle vitality, earth produces his body. These combine in order to produce man. When there is harmony, there is life. Without harmony, there is no life."[1] We should notice here the harmony of body and mind was conceived on the metaphysical level.

This idea that the Heaven contributed to human essence and the earth contributed to human body had a great impact on the later Huanglao texts, such as the *Huinanzi* (淮南子), in which we find the term "*qu xian bi lei*" (取象比類), basic to the methodology of TCM. In fact, the idea of *qu xiang bi lei* was based on this notion of unity between ontology and analogy and the intimate relation between human and Heaven it entailed. As we read in the chapter *Yaolue* 要略 of the *Huainanzi*, summarizing succinctly the discourse developed in the *Jingsheng Xun* 精神訓:

"*The Jingsheng (Subtle Spirit) is that from which human life comes from originally, and also that by which the body in its from and bones and nine holes got enlightened with intelligence. It appropriates its original image (qu xiang) from Heaven, to be combined with blood and breath, therefore human is joyful or anger happens in analogy (bi lei) with the weather's wind and rain, is bright or dark as the change of day and night, winter and*

---

1 The *Guanzi*, p.271

summer. The spirit is capable of discerning the trace of sameness and differences, manage the crucial moment of movement and rest, so as to return to the Origin of its nature and life, to nurture lovingly its Subtle Spirit, to calm and pacify its bodily soul and psychic soul, never allow its authentic self to be changed by external things, while keeping closely to the dwelling of emptiness (xu) and non-being (wu)."[1]

In the *Jingshenxun*, it was made clear that the Subtle Spirit (*jingshen* spirit), which replaced now the Subtle Vital Energy (*jingqi*), was what human beings received from Heaven, and the body was what they inherit from the earth. In this analogical and organist thinking, *"the lungs manifest mainly through the eyes, the kidney through the nose, the gall through the mouth, the liver through the ears, the external as appearance and the internal as the inner reality,...therefore the human head is round, imaging thereby Heaven's form; while human feet are square, imaging the form of the earth. Heaven has its four seasons, five elements, nine divisions, three hundred and sixty six days, while human beings also have four limbs, five organs, nine holes, three hundred sixty six bone sections. Heaven has its weather conditions such as windy, rainy, cold and warm, while human being also has his/her like, dislike, joy and anger. Therefore the gall is like the cloud, the lungs are like the air, the liver is like the wind, the kidney is like the rain, the spleen is like the thunder, so as to take part in the third component of Heaven and earth, while the mind serves as the master."*[2]

This text illustrates very well my affirmation that CTM's methodology, in particular that of *qu xian bi lei*, was conceptually and theoretically founded on Huanglao Daoist philosophy. Indeed, the appropriation of analogical and organist image/ meaning/classification from nature and its manifestations allow the application of the concepts of *qi*, *yin* and *yang*, five elements, etc to the understanding of human body/mind's functions and dysfunctions, and to see the holistic relation between all organs and their intimate interaction with natural environment. Also, in its etiological analysis, the causes of diseases are usually attributed to either externally affected (by in-adaptation to natural change, poison or virus affection) or as internally harmed (by emotions and desires).

---

1 The *Huainanzi* 淮南子, with commentaries by Gao Yu, Taipei: World Book Company, 1985, pp. 370-377. My English translation.
2 Ibid., p.100. My English translation.

Body/Mind and the Technique of Heart

In the *Neiye*, body and mind were not two separate entities. This is to say there was no dualism in Huanglao Daoist view of body and mind. On the contrary, they were always mentioned together as "Mind and Its body" (*xin zhi xin* 心之形), taking thereby the mind as the agent of the body/mind complex. It was supposed that, the mind/body in its natural state was full of *jingqi* and thereby maintained its life, in growing and fulfilling its functions spontaneously. Its loss of the *jingqi* was supposed to be caused by emotional disturbance such as anxiety, joy, happy, anger, desire, and profit. When one was able to get rid of these emotional disturbances, the mind was able to return to its own resources:

"*The Mind's inner reality is benefited by rest and quiet. Avoid being harassed or confused, and its harmony will naturally be complete…It's ever so that Dao has no fixed place to stay. Yet in a good mind it will be peacefully settled. The mind quiescent, and the vital force well managed, the Dao can then be made to stay.*"[1]

To show the agency of the mind, in the *Xinshu* (Technique of Heart) it was said clearly that the relation between body and mind was in analogy with that between a King and his ministers, and the mind should be in control of the movement of the body soberly, like the king of his subjects with non-action (*wuwei* 無為). If the mind was in a state of *no-action*, it could be void, still and one, thereby capable of controlling different members of the body knowingly and discerningly.

"*The relation of mind to body is like the position of a king. Nine holes of our body, just like the officials, have each their own function. If mind is dwelling in the Tao, then all nine holes follow their own principles of function. If the mind is full of desires, then the eyes could not see colors, the ears can not hear sound. Therefore, if the person on high goes astray from the Dao, then the persons under him loose their operations. Do not walk for horse, so that it could unfold its own forces; do nor fly for birds, so that it can exhaust its own ; don't move before things come, so that you can observe its principle.*"[2]

The concept of non-action, according to the early Daoists, meant the universal action of the Dao, without any bias, any particular preferences.

---

1 The *Guanzi*, p.269
2 The *Guanzi*, p.219

However, now it was changed to the state of calm and quiet that the mind (or the king) kept for itself/himself, in letting the body organs or the ministers do by themselves their proper actions in service of him. Therefore, we can tell that, for the Huanglao Daosit, the concept of non-action meant two things. Negatively speaking, it meant not to act before things arrived by themselves, so as to observe their principle of happening. Positively speaking, it meant that the mind, like the king, should be in a state of void, still and unity, which allowed it to be able to control the movement of the body, by being still and calm, deprived of all subjective desire and preference and to follow the formlessness of the Heavenly Dao.

Here the *Inner Working* touched upon the problem of the mind's agency. It was the mind that served as the agent, directing and controlling the body in reducing all desires and emotions. We read,

"When my mind is well regulated, my sense organs are also well regulated. When my mind is at ease, my sense organs are also at ease. That which regulates them is mind; that which sets them at ease is the mind. The mind therefore contains an inner mind. This is to say that in the mind there is again another mind. For this mind, the intention comes before language. The process is like this, there is first the intention, then expression into tangible forms; after tangible forms, there is language. It's by language that we manage[people and things], and it's by way of management that things become regulated. Without regulation there will doom to be disorder. Disorder will certainly bring people and things to death."[1]

The theory of self-cultivation in the *Guanzi* was called "the technique of managing one's heart" (治心之術), abbreviated as "technique of heart" (心術 *xinshu*) or as the inner working (內業 *neiye*) of the mind. This was an art of self-cultivation or life praxis through which one could reduce the negative impact of desires and emotions and keep oneself in the state of calm and quiet so as to make the mind the dwelling of the Dao. If the heart was to be managed by the technique of self-control, it presupposed that human heart might be hindered by emotions, desires and prejudices from attaining the Dao. Therefore, in order to obtain the Dao, one should first of all keep one's heart void (*xu* 虛) and still (*jing* 靜). Since the Dao of Heaven was void, and the Dao of earth was still, therefore, human mind, when void, calm and still, could realize the true nature of Heaven and earth.

---

1 The *Guanzi*, p.270

When void, one's mind did not store, did not query, did not presuppose anything, did not deliberate. When still, human mind calmed itself down and its Qi was thereby well arranged so as to welcome the dwelling of the Dao. These two techniques presuppose Oneness, which meant a sort of mental or spiritual concentration, on the Dao itself of courses, so as not to get astray or deviant from the Dao. These techniques discussed by Huanglao Daoists might have well influenced Xunzi, the last greatest Confucian of Warring States, who interpreted it and integrated it into his own epistemology.

The idea of calming down one's mind in regards to the influence of desires and emotions so as to obtain wisdom was not limited to Huanglao Daoism. For example, Plato, in the *Republic*, where he discussed the training of the future philosopher-king, said that, *"When he has quieted both spirit and appetites, he arouses his third part in which wisdom resides and thus takes his rest; you know that it is then that he best grasps reality."*[1]

In the context of Huanglao Daoist ontology/cosmology, human mind was considered both as the locus of the Dao's dwelling and the agent that managed human desire and purified itself by using various methods. The mind, as the locus of Dao's dwelling, when calm, quiet and purified, was able to receive the Dao and becomes Its dwelling. The mind as an agent of actions, when having its emotions and desires well tempered and under control, would be able to meet the Subtle Qi and performed with its overwhelming power. However, there was no dualism between mind and body. On the contrary, human life lived on the harmonious unity of body and mind.

Practical Methodology

Under the basic conceptual framework explained in the above, the *Inner Working* also discussed some practical methods and the relation between different methods of nurturing life, such as meditation, cultural activities, eating and physical exercise to be discussed in the following.

---

1 Plato, *Republic*, IX, 572a-b

1. Meditation

Meditation was most basic to all Daoist practical methodology, not only because it had the function of reducing desires and emotions and their negative impact, and thereby reducing the possibilities of getting internally harmed, but also because of the good occasion thus offered, when deeply practiced, to rejoin the Subtle Vital Energy and to obtain enlightenment from it. We read,

"If you can run your qi in a marvelous way, myriad things will be complete in your mind. Can you run you qi as such? Can you concentrate you bodily soul and psychic soul in unity? Can you stop your floating thoughts? Can you cease all other external activities? Rather than seeking it in others, can you obtain it within yourself? Mediate, and meditate again, and again, [After such effort of meditation], even if you can not get it through, ghost and spirit will help you through. Indeed, it's not because of their power, but because you have thereby reached the supreme Subtle Qi."[1]

In this text, we find an insisting demand on doing meditation, a demand addressed in particular to the King and political leaders, that they meditate and meditate again and again, the effort of which, when coming up to the state of effortlessness, in a total spiritual concentration, would be able to achieve enlightenment by gathering within oneself all the power of the Subtle Vital Energy (*jingqi*).

2. Therapeutic function of Cultural activities

Huanglao Daoist also absorbed some methods of self-cultivation from Confucianism, in particular as to the positive function of cultural activities, when having conversation with the Confucians in the Jixia Academy. Like the Confucians, they emphasized also the use of poetry, music, and ritual practices and the ethical attitude of respect in their function to reduce the negative impact of desires and emotions, all in putting in priority Daoist concept of "quietude" by saying that "Quietude in side, respect outside". Unlike Confucians who treated poetry, music and ritual practice as object of learning, in stead, Huanglao Daoist used them as practical methods for reducing desires and emotions. We read,

---

[1] The *Guanzi*, p.271

"It is ever so that man's life, is certain to depend on equilibrium and uprightness. Its loss is certainly caused by joy and anger, sorrow and anxiety. Thus, to stop anger, nothing is better than poetry. To rid of sorrow, nothing is better than music. To moderate music, nothing is better than ritual. To preserve the rule of propriety, nothing is better than respect. To preserve the respect, nothing is better than quiescence. Inwardly quiescent and outwardly respectful, people will be able to return to their true nature. And your nature will be greatly stabilized."[1]

3. Eating and Physical Exercise

As to method of eating, the *Neiye* proposed the middle way of eating between gorging and abstention, calling it the "harmonious moderation" in view of bodily health and nurturing life. It analyzed also the relation between eating and physical exercises, in saying that,

"As to the Way of eating, excessive gorging will harm your qi and your body will not prosper. Excessive abstention will dry up your bones, and the blood congeal. The middle way between gorging and abstention is called harmonious moderation. It provides a dwelling for the essence and the birth of knowledge."[2]

The *Neiye* discussed also the relation between eating and physical exercises, saying that after one was too full in eating, one should make faster physical exercise, otherwise the *qi* would not be able to extend properly to the end of four limbs, thus putting the practice of eating, physical exercise and nurturing of life into very close relation.

4. Joyfulness of existence

By discussing matters such as eating and moving about, Huanglao Daoist life praxis was to be realized in everyday life. The principles that one had to follow were temperance, regularity, balance and joyfulness. Above all these, one should encourage one's own mental joyfulness. As the *Neiye* put it:

"Human life should be in a positive state of joyfulness. When it is in anxiety it loses its principle. When angry, it loses its beginnings. When under the impact of anxiety, sorrow, happy and anger, there is no place for

---

1 The *Guanzi*, p.272
2 The *Guanzi*, p.272

Dao. Therefore when you have love and desire, calm them down. When you encounter chaotic situations, rectify it immediately."[1]

This emphasis on la joie d'existence has a great impact on all Daoist literature in dealing with the topic of nurturing life. For example, Shi Tianji (石天基), in his A Song for Getting Rid of Illness, said that, *"The illness comes when one is not in state of joy. When one gets ill, one has to try with all efforts to make oneself happy. When one is happy, illness will be gone. Mental illness needs mental medicine. To be happy is the mental medicine for longevity."*[2] Under the influence of Huanglao Daoism, all the later Daoists, both philosophical and religious, tended to keep a happy and optimist vision of life. We can find, for example, this principle of joyfulness in the earliest Religious Daoist classics, the Taipingjing 太平經, also under the influence of Huanglao Daoism, the following important text:

"To govern body with joyfulness to keep in good form... What is the function of joyfulness for Dao? In fact, to be joyful could harmonize yin and yang, everything when done in quietude, could bring human beings to the root of Dao. Therefore, joyfulness is effected by the good energy and essence in Heaven and earth, through which one could attain the divine enlightenment. Therefore calm could bring forth light, and light is expecting the divine. When one could communicate with the divine and to be near to Dao, then one is qualified to longevity."[3]

From Huanglao Doaism to Religious Daoism, the principle of joyfulness had been emphasized as most important principle for a life of sanity, which was considered as based on a harmonious cosmic and religious foundation, to be practiced with quietude and calmness.

Conclusion

Historically speaking, Huanglao Daoism's concepts of Dao, Qi and Body/Mind relation should have laid the philosophical foundation of Tradi-

---

1 The *Guanzi*, p.272
2 Shi Tianji, "*A Song for Getting Rid of Illness*"(却病歌) quoted in *Taoist Methods of Keeping A Sane Life(Daojia Yangsheng Shu)*, edited by Y.T.Chen, T.W.Lee and C.Y.Liu, Shanghai: Fudan University Press, 1992, p.512
3 This method is entitled "method of discarding calamity through being joyful", see *Critical Edition of Taiping Ching*, edited by Wang Ming, Vol. 1., Beijing: Zhonghua Bookstore, 1960, pp.13-14

tional Chinese Medicine. The methodology of nurturing life (*yangsheng*) and cultivating mind/heart *(xiuxin)*, which preciously combined the bodily health with mental self-cultivation, as developed in the Huanglao texts such as the *Neiye* and the *Xinshu*, were most basic for a Chinese concept of preventive medicine. In fact, in TCM, preventive medicine is more important than curative medicine. As the *Shuwen* (素問 Basic Questions)of *Huandi Neijing* (黃帝內經 Inner Classics of Yellow Emperor) put it well, "The sage does not cure the already ill. He cures all prior to illness. He does not govern things already in disorder. He governs things before they come into disorder. "[1], and that "If one manage to avoid timely those deluding poisons and harmful wind, and lead a life of contentedness, void and freedom, keeping one's inner Spirit intact, where does any disease would come?[2]

Even so, when so many people get sick, they should be cured, which means that curative medicine is equally important, sometimes more needy and even more urgent. There, the role of the doctor is to help people out of their suffering, as an act of humanity and compassion.

---

1 The *Huangdi Neijing, Shuwen(*Basic Questions of the Inner Classics of Yellow Emperor, Taipei: National Institute of Chinese Medicine, 1979, p.11. My English translation.
2 Ibid., p.7

Lan Fengli

Globalization of TCM: Cultural Differences between TCM and Western Medicine

The thesis discusses cultural differences between traditional Chinese medicine (TCM) and Western medicine from the linguistic and philosophical aspects, the unique values of TCM, and advances some suggestions in the process of globalization of TCM.

Both transmission of TCM to the West and dissemination of Western medicine in China started in the Ming dynasty (16th-17th centuries). Some missionaries taught and spread religion by practicing Western medicine; meanwhile, they introduced TCM curiously, esp. their own experiences in TCM, to the West. Over 300 years passed by. At present, TCM and Western medicine actually coexist no matter in China or in the West. TCM is not only a special medical system with distinctive national features of China, but is also a medical system for the mankind of the whole world.

Both TCM and Western medicine are "scientific systems of studying life processes of the human being and prevention and treatment of diseases".[1] It is thus clear that they share at least 3 common characters, i.e. the same object – life processes of the human being; the same goal – to prevent and treat diseases; and both are members of "scientific systems". But, TCM bears strong humane characteristics; while Western medicine, esp. modern Western medicine, has typical features of modern Western science. What are the cultural differences between the two medical systems? How do the differences influence the dissemination of TCM in the West, or even globalization of TCM?

1. Cultural Differences between TCM and Western Medicine

A leading authority on Chinese herbal medicine, Dr. Yakazu Domei, lists the following differences between TCM and Western Medicine:[2]

---

1 Xia Zheng-Nong. Sea of Words. Shanghai: Shanghai Dictionary Press, 2002: 2006.
2 www.tcmhelp.com/Theory/3.htm

	Chinese Medicine	Western Medicine
1.	Philosophical	Scientific
2.	Synthetic	Analytical
3.	Holistic	Topical
4.	Internal	Surgical
5.	Conformational	Heteropathic
6.	Empirical	Theoretical
7.	Hygienic	Preventive
8.	Individualized	Socialized
9.	Preventive	Bacteriological
10.	Experiential	Experimental
11.	Humoral	Cellular
12.	Subjective	Objective
13.	Natural sources	Synthetic analogy

I will talk about the cultural differences between TCM and Western Medicine from linguistic and philosophical aspects.

1.1 Linguistic Differences

"Language is the outcome of culture. Language of a nation is the general reflection of the culture of the nation; but we can also say that language is a part of the culture, and that culture and language have developed together for thousands of years."[1]

1.1.1 Ideographic Writing, Phonetic Writing, and Thinking Ways

1.1.1.1 Ideographic Writing and Thinking Ways of TCM

Chinese characters are the only ideographic writing (as opposed to phonetic writing) which has been preserved for over 3,000 years. As early as in the years of 100-121 A.D., Xu Shen 许慎 of the Eastern Han Dynasty wrote and compiled the first systematic dictionary with complete collection of characters, comprehensive analysis of the shape, pronunciation and meanings as well as scientific arrangement: *The Origin of Chinese Cha-*

---

1 Quoted from A Secondary Source: He Yu-Min. Differences, Perplexity and Selection: A Comparative Study of Chinese Medicine and Western Medicine. Shenyang: Shenyang Press, 1990: 149.

racters (shuo wen jie zi,《说文解字》). He systematically expounded the theoretical system of the structures of Chinese characters in an all-round way for the first time: the six scripts or the six categories, i.e. *xiangxing* 象形, *zhishi* 指事, *huiyi* 会意, *xingsheng* 形声, *zhuanzhu* 转注 and *jiajie* 假借, and analyzed the structures and meanings of over 9,000 Chinese characters according to the system. Although *The Origin of Chinese Characters* presents and exists in the form of a dictionary, its academic value is far beyond that of the dictionaries in the common sense.

After investigating the authors and their formation times of *The Origin of Chinese Characters* and *Huang Di's Inner Classic*, I have found that it is very possible that the former is influenced by the latter. The following conclusions are reached through comparing and analyzing thinking ways, philosophical conception, and knowledge of human anatomy, disease and treatment in them: ① The knowledge of TCM contained in *The Origin of Chinese Characters* is in direct line of succession with the *Inner Classic*; ② The universal and eco-medical thinking ways of "Heaven-Earth-Human being" in them are cut from the same cloth; ③ The theories of qi, yin-yang, and the five phases, the theoretical foundation of the *Inner Classic*, can be traced back to their sources through *The Origin of Chinese Characters* which expounds the original meanings of them by analyzing their structures ; ④ *The Origin of Chinese Characters* traces back to characters' origin and original meanings through analyzing their structures, therefore, it is a very helpful and important book to study and read the *Inner Classic*, and to probe into the origin of TCM as well.[1]

Let's take *qi* 气 as an example. *The Origin of Chinese Characters·Qi Section* states that "*Qi* refers to thin, floating clouds. The character 气 is a pictographic character."[2] The character 气 in *Jia Gu Wen* 甲骨文, the inscriptions on bones or tortoise shells of the Shang Dynasty (c. 16th-11th century B.C.), was written as "川", which resembles air current, evaporating and rising, whose image is just like cloud, will disappear very soon and become invisible. Therefore, *qi* is invisible and formless, exists everywhere,

---

1 Lan Fengli. Influence of *Huang Di's Inner Classic* on *The Origin of Chinese Characters*. Chinese Journal of Medical History, 2006, 36(4):201-205.
2 Written by Xu Shen [Han], Annotated by Duan Yu-Cai [Qing]. The Origin of Chinese Characters with Annotations. Shanghai: Shnaghai Ancient Books Press, 1988: 20.

can be gathered into a form, for instance, *qi* can be condensed into water. *Qi* at this moment referred to air or vapor.

Soon afterwards, the *qi* which surrounds and congests the space of the human being was abstracted into the *qi* which bears a material meaning in philosophical sense. Philosophers of materialism of the Spring Autumn and Warring States Period (770-221B.C.) believed that *qi* is the basic material constituting the world, and that everything in the universe comes into being by the movement and mutation of *qi*. For example, *Book of Changes • Section Xi Ci,* (Zhou Yi •Xi Ci,《周易•系辞》) states that "everything is transformed and generated by the enshrouding [qi] of the heaven and earth".

Later on, ancient Chinese medical experts introduced "*qi*" into the medical field at the right moment. And then, "*qi*" became a medium or bridge between the natural philosophy of the pre-Qin days (i.e. before 221 B.C. when the First Emperor of Qin united China) and Chinese medicine. The concept of "*qi*" gradually formed in TCM.

In the time of *Huangdi's Inner Classic*, "*qi*" is regarded not only as the basic material constituting the world, but also as the basic material constituting the human being which can be transformed into blood, essence, and body fluid, etc., and the normal functional activities of the life which is governed by "qi" is known as *Shen* or spirit.[1]

It is thus evident that the shape of a Chinese character is directly related to its meaning, and both integrate into a unity. The formation of a Chinese character, an organic whole of the shape and the meaning, is one-step made following the rule of nature, reflecting the direct communication between and integration of the subject and the object. The formation also implies an important thinking way, i.e. thinking in terms of images. Integration of the subject and the object is a thread running through the Chinese traditional culture and science, on the basis of which the unification of the Heaven and Human being (tian ren he yi, 天人合一) constitutes the foundation of the Chinese traditional culture and sciences. Thinking in terms of images is a traditional thinking way of the Chinese nation, and whose process, methods, and rules make up the thinking in terms of im-

---

1 Lan Fengli. The Origin of *Qi, Yin-Yang* and *Wu Xing* as Chinese Medical Concepts and Their Translation. In Wallner, Kubiena & Jandl (eds.), Understanding Traditional Chinese Medicine [C]. Frankfurt a.M.: Peter Lang, 2009.

ages and reasoning from analogy (qu xiang bi lei, 取象比类), the framework of the Chinese traditional culture and sciences.

Developed on the basis of the ideographic writing, Chinese characters and their meanings are quite stable and conservative, which greatly promotes the development of the thinking in terms of images and reasoning from analogy of ancient TCM experts. Then such a thinking way was set up in the *Huang Di's Inner Classic* and has greatly influenced TCM experts of the later generations.

The ideographic writings of yin-yang 阴阳, *wu xing, or five phases* 五行, *jing or essence* 精, and *qi*, the extensive analogical and abundant imagery thinking examples in the *Huang Di's Inner Classic*, and criticism, proofreading, annotations for characters from the aspects of the "shape", "pronunciation", and "meaning" in the ancient medical classics made in the Ming (1368-1644 A.D.) and Qing Dynasties (1644-1911 A.D.), all demonstrate the far-reaching influences of the ideographic thinking way on the development of TCM.

1.1.1.2 Phonetic Writing, and Thinking Ways of Western Medicine

Phonetic writing (as opposed to ideographic writing) is the most common writing in the world. English, German, French, Spanish, Portuguese, etc. are all phonetic writing, but are different languages composed by the same Latin alphabet. Let's take English as a case in point.

The shapes of the English words are directly related to the pronunciations, but have nothing to do with the meanings or the external images of concrete things. That is to say, in phonetic writing, the shape is separate and independent from the meaning, and the meaning comes from man-made prescript outside the shape, which indicates that the formation of a word of the phonetic writing is composed of two steps: first, building its shape (spelling of alphabets); second, defining its meaning (linguistic rules or grammar). The understanding of the meanings of words is based on the sense of hearing, thus jumping out the thinking frame of the visual sense of the concrete images of things, then providing a bigger possibility for logic thinking based on the abstraction, finally forming thinking traditions of abstract inference, conceptual thinking, categorization, and trying to make an objective judgment to the world.

This is really indeed the case. The formation of phonetic writing reflects its two important characteristics: tool (alphabet) and abstraction (linguistic rules). Every tool is made to have a certain function according to human beings' specific aim or intention, thus becoming a medium of connection between human beings and the nature, and so interrupting the natural direct communication between them. Tool plays a vital role in the Western culture, esp. in the natural sciences, where it is standardized and systematized, and the experimental research approach characterized by the use of various tools is set up. Actually, the alphabet is the mother of various tools. The thinking way corresponding to the experimental research approach is abstraction. The rule of abstraction is logic, while linguistic rules or grammar is an embryonic form of logic.[1]

The emergence of tool reflects the relationship between the subject and the object, i.e., the separation and opposition of them (man remakes the nature). The abstraction pays more attention to being analytical, logical, and restricts imagination. The tool and abstraction become the foundation of the Western culture and sciences and of the natural sciences (including the Western medicine) in particular. The Western natural sciences manifest in two opposite ways or two edges, which have been realized by more and more people as time goes by. The two edges lie in that environmental pollution and ecological imbalance, the repay of the nature to the human beings, always accompany the process of human conquering and remaking nature. As regards to the Western medicine, the two edges lie in that severe side effects, drug resistance, and effect being temporary always accompany the notable therapeutic effects.

1.1.2 Chinese Medical Terminology and Western Medical Terminology

Undoubtedly, no matter the language of TCM or the language of Western medicine is a kind of technical language. Modern terminologists define a "technical language" as a form of any given language that is used by people involved in a special field and that has a "terminology", i.e., a set of expressions not used in the common language or, as is often the case, expressions that are used in a different or more specific way than in the common language.

---

1 Wang Zhen-Hua. Theoretical Difference between TCM and Western Medicine on the Basis of Linguistics: Modernization of TCM. China Journal of Traditional Chinese Medicine. 2001: 16 (6): 5

A popular misconception about technical terms is that they are words used *exclusively* by specialists. *In actual fact, technical terms in most disciplines largely, if not mostly, come from the common language.* Any language only has a certain number of words, and new terms are usually combinations of existing lexical items. Many terms are completely indistinguishable in form from expressions in the common language although they are more specific in meaning. The process whereby common language expressions are given more specific or metaphorical meanings in the technical contexts is called "terminologization". *The modern terminological observation that technical terms are largely derived from the common language is reflected clearly both in TCM and Western medicine.* Those acquainted with the language of TCM are aware that most of the characters they come across in Chinese medical texts are used in the common language. And most of the Western medical terms are combinations of morphemes of Latin or Greek. Actually, about 10,000 Latin or Greek words came into English during the Renaissance Period and finally became a part of English vocabulary.

Actually, both TCM terminology and Western medical terminology can be classified into three levels: ① words and expressions for everyday use; ② specialized terms of their own; and ③ original terms of their own.

1.1.2.1 Three Levels of Chinese Medical Terminology

Both Wiseman and Unschuld advocated classifying the basic Chinese medical terminology into two categories: one comprises of words and expressions for everyday use, e.g., 头 head, 脚 foot, 胸 chest, 腹 abdomen, 心 heart, 肝 liver, 血 blood; the other is composed of specialized TCM terms extended from the common language and formed through metaphor or analogy, e.g., 窍 orifice, 穴 point or hole, 正 upright, 邪 evil, 营 nutrient, 卫 defense, 命门 life gate, 督脉 the governing vessel, 三焦 triple passage or triple burner or triple energizer.[1] [Note: The character 焦, as a common character, does mean "burnt" or "charred", but as a medical term, it means "passage or space within the body" that is well explained in some specialized Chinese dictionaries]

---

1 Wiseman, Nigel. Translation and Transmission of Chinese Medicine in the West. Medicine and Philosophy. 2001, 22(7): 51-54.

According to my understanding of Chinese medical terminology, esp. of *the Origin of Chinese Characters*, I think that Chinese medical terminology can be classified into 3 levels. The first level is made up of *words and expressions from the common language*, e.g., some body parts like 心 heart, 肝 liver, 脾 spleen, 肺 lungs, 肾 kidneys, 鼻 nose, 目 eyes, 耳 ears, 头 head, 脚 foot, 胸 chest, 腹 abdomen, 血 blood; some disease names like 霍乱 cholera, 麻疹 measles, 麻风 leprosy, 疟疾 malaria, 癫痫 epilepsy; some climatic pathogenic factors like 风 wind, 寒 cold, 湿 dampness, 燥 dryness, 火 fire; some symptoms like 发热 fever, 头痛 headache, 痛 pain, 咳嗽 cough, 心悸 palpitation, 健忘 forgetfulness, 头晕目眩 dizziness, 呕吐 vomiting, 恶心 nausea, 泄泻 diarrhea, 便秘（不更衣）constipation. The second level constitutes *specialized Chinese medical terms from daily words and expressions formed through metaphor or analogy*, e.g., 藏 depots or viscera, 府 palaces or bowels, 经 meridian or channel, 络 collateral or network vessel, 窍 orifice, 穴 point or hole, 正 upright, 邪 evil, 营 nutrient, 卫 defense, 督脉 the governing vessel, 任脉 the controlling vessel, 三焦 the triple energizer or *san jiao*, 命门 life gate, etc. *which usually bear historical, cultural, and medical values at the same time.* The third level comprises of *original Chinese medical terms, e.g., some pictophonetic characters* such as 疝, 疸, 痈, 疡, 痔, 痿, 痹, etc. in *The Origin of Chinese Characters • Disease Section.*

1.1.2.2 Three Levels of Western Medical Terminology

Dr. Wiseman roughly classified the Western medical terminology into 3 levels and distinguished them as well. The first level constitutes *borrowings from the common language*, e.g., fever, chill, cough, cold, hiccough, headache, pain, tenderness, soreness, palpitations, bleeding, hot flushes, forgetfulness, dizziness, vomiting, blindness, jaundice, deafness, nausea, emaciation, diarrhea, constipation, goiter, sores, corn, sty, boil, measles, mumps, and fracture. These words, commonly used by doctors, are known to all speakers and denote conditions that can be identified by most normal adults. The second level comprises *terms devised by modern medicine to describe certain technical concepts*: conjunctivitis, anemia, hypertension, paranasal sinusitis, trichomoniasis, arteriosclerosis, optic atrophy, hyperchlorhydria, coronary thrombosis, glomerulonephritis hematoma, cerebrovascular ischemia. Although some of these words (such as anemia, hypertension and conjunctivitis) may be familiar to and even used by non-experts, the conditions they denote cannot be diagnosed by the non-experts with the medical precision. These terms *reflect knowledge that lies at a long distance from lay understanding*. Between these two levels is *a third comprising terms of medical origin* that do not require any specialist knowledge or instrumentation to understand or identify, e.g., enuresis, lochia, pharynx, larynx, dysphagia, strangury, scrofula, tumor, fistula, miliaria, macule, papule, and diphtheria.[1]

I think that the terms of the first level are actually from *words and expressions for everyday use*, that of the second level are *specialized terms of Western medicine*, and that of the third level are *original terms of Western medicine*.

1.1.2.3 Remarks

In the course of transmission and exchange of medical cultures, linguistic contact is a forerunner of the contact of different medical cultures. Language, an essential medium, is the carrier of the medical knowledge. The transmission and exchange between different medical cultures will first manifest in the terminology. The foreign terminology comes to be the "envoy" of the different medical cultures. Generally speaking, a foreign medical culture is introduced and disseminated by translating the foreign medical terminology. The translated terminology gradually integrates into the native language, finally becomes an organic part of the mainstream medical culture of the nation proper.

The history of translation and dissemination of Western medicine in China shows that the Western medical terminology and culture are very closely associated with each other, just like the shadow following the person. It also took a very long time for the formation of standard Chinese translation of Western medical terminology in China. In the early stage of translation and dissemination of Western medicine in China, for example, translation of the term "scarlet fever" had been very confusing, which had many different translations such as 红热症，红疹，疹子热病，痧病，花红热症，猩红热，etc.

---

1 Wiseman, Nigel. The Translation of Chinese Medical Terminology. English-Chinese & Chinese-English Dictionary of Chinese Medicine, Changsha: Hunan Science and Technology Press, 1996: 67.

It can be seen from the history and reality of translating Western medicine into Chinese that the first and third levels of the Chinese medical terms have been successfully used to express Western medical knowledge, and that using the second level of Chinese medical terms, which carry the most distinctive TCM knowledge, to translate specialized terms of Western medicine, has produced serious confusions or even mistakes. Here are two examples:

① Translating "typhoid" into 伤寒 Typhoid refers to "infection of the intestine caused by *Salmonella typhi* in food and water"[1] manifesting in fever, diarrhea, even bloody stool; while 伤寒 is a specialized Chinese medical term, bears two meanings in TCM: in a broad sense, 伤寒, cold-induced disease, is a general term for various externally contracted febrile diseases, as stated in the *Plain Questions·Discourse on Febrile Diseases* (su wen·re lun, 《素问•热论》) "今夫热病者，皆伤寒之类也"; in a narrow sense, 伤寒, cold affection, refers to a condition caused by cold, manifesting in chills and fevers, absence of sweating, headache, floating and tense pulse, as stated in the *Classic of Difficult Issues* (nan jing, 《难经·五十八难》"伤寒有五：有中风，有伤寒，有湿温，有热病，有温病，其所苦各不同". Later on, some translators rendered 伤寒 in Chinese medicine back into "typhoid". Such a translation has confused the differences between "typhoid" in Western medicine and 伤寒 in Chinese medicine, thus causing misunderstanding or even misleading the readers.

② Translating "surgery" into 外科学 Surgery refers to "treatment of a disease or disorder which requires an operation to cut into or to remove or to manipulate tissue or organs or parts"[2]; while 外科学 in TCM refers to a specialty which studies the causes, pathogenesis, and treatments of the diseases on the body surface.[3] Many TCM undergraduates or even doctorate candidates, and some translators translate 外科学 in TCM into "Surgery". Actually, 外科学 in TCM should be translated into "external medicine" for the real "surgery" in TCM declined long ago since Hua Tuo died in 208 A.D.

---

1 Collin, P.H. Dictionary of Medicine. Beijing: Foreign Language Teaching and Research Press, 2001: 613, 571.
2 Collin, P.H. Dictionary of Medicine. Beijing: Foreign Language Teaching and Research Press, 2001: 613, 571.
3 Li Jing-Wei, et al. A Concise Dictionary of Chinese Medicine. Beijing: China Press of Traditional Chinese Medicine:301.

We should draw some lessons from the above mentioned translation examples that the second level of Western medical terms should not be used to translate and express the specialized Chinese medical terms. For example, although 风火眼 in TCM and "acute conjunctivitis" in Western medicine actually refer to the same disease, it is ill-advised to translate 风火眼 into "acute conjunctivitis" for such a translation must confuse cultural differences between the two medical systems, and fail to produce such association of the cause (pathogenic wind-fire) and therapeutic method (coursing wind and clearing fire) with the translation "acute conjunctivitis", thus destroying the independency, wholeness and systematicness of the theoretical system of TCM.

An interesting issue to be addressed is that some disease names in the *Plain Questions (su wen)* may be of foreign origin. Here are some examples: *li lai* 疠癞: 疠 , whose ancient pronunciation is *ljadh* or *rjats*, and 癞 , whose ancient pronunciation is *ladh* or *rats* , the initial consonants come closer to those of the three most popular ancient European terms for *leprosy*, one might speculate about an association of *li* and *lai* with *leuke, lepra, and e-lephantiasis* ; *huo luan* 霍乱 , the compound *huo luan* does not correspond to the graphic structure of the vast majority of ancient Chinese disease terms, while its ancient pronunciation **hwak* luan* was formed to reflect in ancient Chinese the sound of the term *cholera* used along the travel routes from regions where the Greek term was in use to the Far East to designate a particularly violent type of diarrhea; *fei xiao* 肺消, whose ancient pronunciation is **phjats*sjaw,* literally "lung wasting", could be a rendering into Chinese of the ancient Greek term *phtisis* or lung *phtisis,* which has exactly the same meaning; xiao ke 消渴 , wasting/melting and thirst, a label used to this day for diabetes, is a compound ideally suited to signify two obvious symptoms of the disease. An identical meaning was expressed in European antiquity by Aretaios of Cappadochia.[1] Is it purely coincidental? Or there existed medical cultural exchange between the East and the West around the Zhou Dynasty (C. 1100-256 B.C.)? Anyway, these terms all came out far before the modern Western medicine and should be regarded as the terms of the first level. The above

---

1 Unschuld, Paul U. Huang Di Nei Jing Su Wen: Nature, Knowledge, Imagery in An Ancient Chinese Medical Text. Berkeley: University of California Press, 2003: 203-204.

understanding further provides etymological evidence when translating 疠癫, 霍乱, 肺消, 消渴 into *leprosy, cholera, lung wasting, wasting and thirst* respectively.

1.1.3 Medical Classical Chinese and Medical English

First of all, let's look at the two paragraphs about the origin of human life both from the angle of genetics in TCM and Western medicine respectively:

① "人生于地，悬命于天，天地合气，命之曰人。人能应四时者，天地为之父母"（《素问•宝命全形论》）.

Translation: Man is born on the earth, hanging his life to the heaven. The union of celestial qi and terrestrial qi make up a man. Man can adapt himself to the seasons for the Heaven and Earth are his parents. (Plain Questions·Discourse on Protecting Life and Preserving Physical Appearance)

② "Man is metazoon, triploblastic, chordale, vertebrate, pentadactyle, mammalian, eutherian, primate… The outlines of each of his principal system of organs may be traced back, like those of other mammals, to the fishes." (L.A.B.-orradaile)

（译文：人属于后生动物，系五趾，三胚层高级动物，属脊索动物门，脊椎动物亚门，哺乳纲，灵长目……象其它哺乳动物一样，他的每一个器官系统的轮廓可以追溯到鱼类。）[1]

It is thus clear that the Chinese language of the first paragraph is very elegant and beautiful, is composed of four-character or six-character sentences like a poem or a prose, thus pertaining to classical style and bearing some characteristics of humane studies; while the English language of the second paragraph is very rigorous and precise, comprises of technical terms, thus pertaining to technical style and bearing typical features of Western science.

It is well known that the core knowledge of TCM comes from the ancient medical texts in classical style of writing. In fact, the TCM language has been set to "classical style of writing" since the era of *Huang Di's Inner Classic*. Medical classical Chinese is one of "classical styles of writing", a literary style of writing. TCM terminology is polysemous and ambiguous, and medical classical Chinese is very succinct in style and rich in figures

---

1 Hou Wei-Rui. English Styles of Writing. Shanghai: Shanghai Foreign Language Education Press, 1988: 278.

of speech, so the meanings of TCM language tend to be ambiguous and initiate contentions among different schools. The theoretical framework of TCM is extraordinary stable and has almost no breakthrough since *Huang Di's Inner Classic, Classic of Difficult Issues, Shen Nong's Classic of Materia Medica*, and *Treatise on Cold-Induced and Miscellaneous Diseases* came out several thousands of years ago. TCM has been paying excessive attention to wording since the era of the *Inner Classic*, and textual criticism, exegetical studies and annotations of ancient medical classics has been an important academic field of study in TCM up till now, thus reflecting its characteristics of humane and social studies.

As regards to Western medicine, esp. modern Western medicine, it is no doubt that it has been developing with amazing speed and has made many breakthroughs and astonishing achievements in the 19th-21st centuries. "The main reason that the natural sciences have developed more mature than the social sciences is that most of the natural sciences have liberated themselves from the wording disputations and that paying excessive attention to wording has been still spreading unchecked in various ways in the social sciences no matter in the past or nowadays".[1]

1.2 Philosophical Differences

Philosophy, the core of culture and the theoretical thinking of the top level, has been guiding the development of medicine and other sciences. Traditional Western thinking mode is known as analytical thinking, causal thinking, or conceptual thinking[2], on the basis of which the mechanism, reductionism, dichotomy formed and greatly promoted the development of Western medicine. Surgery and organ transplantation medicine have developed on the basis of the mechanism which views the human body as a "machine". On the basis of reductionist ideology or reductionism–that is, it seeks to understand a system by breaking it down into its constituent parts, experimental physiology and cellular biology were founded in the 19th century and molecular biology was founded in the 20th century; influenced by

---

1 Quoted from A Secondary Source: He Yu-Min. Differences, Perplexity and Selection: A Comparative Study of Chinese Medicine and Western Medicine. Shenyang: Shenyang Press, 1990: 170.
2 Fang Ke-Li. A Fusion of Chinese and Western Cultures and Modern Transformation of Chinese Philosophy. Beijing: Commercial Press, 2003: 140-143.

such a thinking, the Western medicine has studied various systems and organs of the body down to cell, to molecule, and to gene in the recent 2 centuries, and constructed a series branches of learning of basic medicine, thus forming the so-called "scientific" Western medicine. Dichotomy, philosophy of a division into two opposite parts–A and Non-A , indicates the separation of the subject and object, of the nature and human being, of the time and space, of the body and mind, of the ontology and epistemology, and so and so forth, guides the treating principle of Western medicine as well which treats a condition using drugs which produce opposite symptoms to those of the condition.

Traditional Chinese thinking mode is known as correlative thinking[1], which originated in the *Book of Changes* and is mainly characterized by explaining dynamic life processes by opposing and complementing as the Yin-Yang Diaphragm suggests. The correlative thinking sees everything in the universe as interdependent and interactive. In TCM, the correlative thinking manifests itself concretely in the yin-yang theory, the five-phase theory, and the visceral image theory, the vessel theory, etc., which evolved in the way of following the features of the heaven and earth (nature) to the human being from concrete to abstract, from structure to function. In TCM, disease is regarded as the result of imbalance or disharmony of yin and yang, and the goal of TCM treatment is to restore the balance for each individual under his or her own unique environment.

Actually, correlative thinking mode of Eastern tradition and causal thinking mode of Western tradition depend on each other and complement to each other, to some extent oppose to each other. More and more scholars in the West have recognized this point.

Compared to the Western philosophical thinking mode, traditional Chinese philosophical thinking mode is not inferior at all, but can be a perfect complement to the Western philosophical thinking. The two traditions should understand each other, respect each other. Only in this way, each tradition can understand its own culture more thoroughly; the two traditions can promote each other and develop together.

---

1 Fang Ke-Li. A Fusion of Chinese and Western Cultures and Modern Transformation of Chinese Philosophy. Beijing: Commercial Press, 2003: 140-143.

2. Unique Values of TCM

2.1 Unique Value of TCM Theories

Most of traditional medical systems declined long ago. But TCM has aroused attention and studies of the world medical circle. What is the reason? Is it due to Chinese medicinals or acupuncture or thousands of years of clinical experiences? No, it is not really the case. The key lies in that TCM has a set of systematic, macrocosmic theory which can effectively guide clinical practice, challenge or even overcome baffling problems of the world medical circle. For example, SARS (Severe Acute Respiratory Syndrome) was so successfully treated in China according to the Warm Disease Theory during its attack in 2003 that experts of World Health Organization (WHO) highly appraised the effects and suggested to improve such clinical experiences to a level of routine treatment; Prof. Deng Tie-Tao (邓铁涛) successfully treated many stubborn diseases such as gravis myoasthenia, atrophic gastritis, hepatitis, cirrhosis, aplastic anemia, lupus erythematosus, etc. according to the Spleen-Stomach Theory; many cases with high fever who failed to respond to antibiotics or antipyretics were successfully cured according to the Theory of Sweet and Warm Medicinals Being Capable of Relieving High Fever.

TCM theories are unique in Chinese sciences and culture and are based on the correlative thinking and holism, therefore, reductionist methodology of the Western scientific approach is not applicable for the study of TCM. For example, White Tiger Decoction is a famous formula for relieving high fever. But Western pharmacological studies found that each ingredient of the formula did not show any effect in relieving fever in experimental animals, which indicates that the reductionist methodology does not work in traditional Chinese pharmacological studies and that traditional Chinese pharmacological studies can not break away from the systematic theory and clinical practice of TCM.

Deng Tie-Tao said, "Microcosmic is a scientific approach, macrocosmic is also a scientific approach. Scientific studies can be done not only based on microcosmic approach, but also can be done on the basis of macrocosmic approach of TCM".[1] "TCM and Western medicine should not repel each other but should complement each other. Integration of micro-

---

1 Bian Shi Ji (A Collection of Distinguished TCM Experts' Papers). Beijing: China Press of Traditional Chinese Medicine, 2001: 4.

cosmic and macrocosmic approaches will produce a more profound theory, and achieve a better therapeutic effect. This is the developmental orientation of post-modern sciences".[1]

2.2 Distinctive Glamour of TCM Therapeutics

TCM has survived the challenge of Western medicine and even advanced to some extent in the 20th-21st centuries mainly for it can effectively treat many diseases. It is well known that most of gynecological disorders such as menstrual disorders, infertility, climacteric syndrome, etc. can be successfully treated by TCM while Western medicine can only provide hormone and surgical operation.

As regards to emergency treatments, *Da Chai Hu* Decoction recorded in *Treatise on Cold-Induced Diseases* (*Shang han lun*, 《伤寒论》) is remarkably effective in treating acute pancreasitis, *Da Jian Zhong* Decoction recorded in *Synopsis of the Golden Chamber* (*Jin Kui Yao Lue*, 《金匮要略》) remarkably effective in treating paralytic intestinal obstruction, puncturing the *Si Feng* points (EX-UE10) remarkably effective in treating intestinal obstruction due to round worms, and so and so forth.

Both history and reality have proved that lemology of TCM also has its own distinctive glamour---TCM has successfully resolved prevention and treatment of various infectious diseases, esp. infectious diseases caused by various viruses, such as encephalitis B, measles complicated with pneumonia, SARS, etc. Besides, TCM can also successfully deal with functional disorders of the nervous, endocrine, and immune systems, diseases of undetermined causes, diseases of complicated causes and pathomechanism, diseases in chronic or recovery stage, and disease prevention and health preservation based on pattern identification and treatment.

2.3 Doctor's Cardinal Humane Care to Patient (medical morality): Different Relationship between Doctor and Patient

In TCM culture, medicine is a kind of benevolent skill, a doctor should be benevolent to the patients, cultivate his morality, love his career, study di-

---

1 Deng Tie-Tao. Correctly Understanding Chinese Medicine. China Newspaper of Chinese Medicine. 2003, (2):17.

ligently, train hard, be conscientious, responsible, modest and prudent, respect his colleagues, which fully reflect in Sun Simiao's *Medical Morality* (or A great doctor should be expert in medical skills and sincere to the patients, da yi jing cheng, 《大医精诚》, the preface of the *Invaluable Prescriptions for Emergencies*, bei ji qian jin yao fang, 《备急千金要方》; Sun Si-Miao, 541or 581~682, a great doctor of the Tang Dynasty).

Sun Si-Miao said, "When the well-qualified doctors treat patients, they should be calm and concentrated without any desire or avarice. First of all, they should have great sympathy for the patients and then be determined to save people from the suffering. When patients come to ask for help, they should not treat them differently by seeing whether they are rich or poor, old or young, beautiful or ugly, enemy or friend, Chinese or foreigner, foolish or wise. They should treat all the patients like their close relatives. When treating patients, they should not think over and over for themselves and pay too much attention to the protection of their own lives. Being qualified doctors, they should regard the patients' suffering as their own and have deep sympathy for them. They should not try to avoid danger if being confronted with it. No matter in daytime or night, winter or summer, no matter they are hungry or thirsty, tired or exhausted, they should treat or save patients heart and soul without any delay or worrying about personal gains or losses. Only by so doing can they become great doctors for people".

3. Globalization of TCM: Opportunity and Challenge

We have to face such a stern reality: Information in English accounted for over 80% of the total information stored in the computers of the world; databases owned by U.S.A. made up over 70% of the globe;[1] the statistics of the United Nations showed that of all the original documents 80% were in English and less than 1% in Chinese; there existed great deficit in the cultural exchange: the works translated from Western languages into Chinese were about 50 to 100 times of the works translated from Chinese into Western languages.[2]

---

1 Yu Ke-Ping. Globalization: Westernization or Chinesization. Beijing: Social Sciences Academic Press, 2002: 4-256.
2 Wang Yue-Chuan. Discovering the East. Beijing Library Press, 2003: 29.

Does globalization mean Westernization, Easternization or similarization or even uniformation? No, globalization should be pluralization. Almost everybody has traveling experience. As a traveler, everyone would like to see something, some place, and some people with distinctive, specialized, and local features. If everywhere is the same someday in the future, the world will be very boring. This is the same as the culture. Standing on the international academic platform, reviewing the history of human beings fighting against diseases, preserving health and prolonging life, we have to realize that TCM is a real gem worth to cherish and to carry on in the unending quest for human health and a long life.

3.1 Standardize Academic Language of TCM

We have to establish the coordinate rules of TCM before opening a dialogue for the cultural exchange of TCM with outside world. First of all, we should strengthen the studies on the standardization of academic language of TCM in the process of translating and introducing TCM works to the West. As Shigeru Omi said, *"Science and civilization have developed because of language.* Likewise, traditional medicine has been developing for thousands of years with its own set of terms. ... Although traditional medicine can be defined with indigenous characters, its terminology should be standardized for modern usage. International standard terminology will greatly expedite scientific communications in traditional societies. *It is the very first step towards the globalization of traditional medicine."*[1]

We should systematize the basic theories, fundamental propositions, core concepts, essential terminology and key words of TCM, make them conformable to each other, then expound and make a comment on them in a rationale way for the purpose of avoiding misunderstanding or misleading the readers in the process of outputting TCM.

We should interpret Chinese medical classics thoroughly with plentiful clinical experiences and modern research results, not just explain the classics word for word.

---

[1] WHO Western Pacific Region. WHO International Standard Terminologies on Traditional Medicine in the Western Pacific Region. Forward. 2007.

It is very important to study the differences between TCM in China (original TCM) and the TCM transmitted in the West in order to learn from each other, bridge the gap and make TCM better known, studied, and appreciated for many years to come no matter in China or in the West.

3.2 Popularize TCM Knowledge Worldwide

It is very important to popularize medical knowledge to the common people, esp. the knowledge of TCM to the young people, in order to let them know the advantages and disadvantages of TCM and Western medicine. Encourage them to see more TCM. According to Wu Yi's (吴仪, Vice Primer of the Government of China) talk on the development of TCM, TCM knowledge in popular language will be written into textbooks of primary and middle schools in China in the near future. The role and position of TCM in the health care system of China is vital in the process of spreading it worldwide.

A cooperation group, which is composed of Chinese and Western scholars of the related fields, should be organized in order to translate and introduce real TCM in a more attractive, readable and "digestive" way in different levels to the corresponding intended readers. For example, the books should be translated or written in a popular style and good language for the common people; for practitioners of TCM, TCM academic language, which preserves the systematicness, independency, and wholeness of the theoretical system of TCM, should be strictly applied; for experts of medical history, the translation should preserve the cultural, historical, and medical values of the original texts; for doctors or researchers of Western medicine, the text should contain more modern research results, or more "evidence-based"; etc.

3.3 Keep Characteristics of TCM and Bring Them into Full Play

As we all know, individualized treatment based on pattern identification is one of the basic characteristics and great vitality of TCM. Therefore, we should study the essence and connotations of pattern identification and treatment; try to discover the relationship among patterns in TCM and physio-chemical indexes, diseases in modern Western medicine; apply modern technology to check the therapeutic effects of TCM, or even invent some new apparatus in the light of TCM theory to check the effects; set up or found a system in the light of TCM theory to assess, approve, and verify research projects or modern studies of TCM.

In the context of globalization, the differences of TCM from Western medicine should be highlighted in almost all aspects. For example, the appearance and inner design of the TCM clinics or hospitals should reflect TCM cultural features such as by using yin-yang diaphragm, popularizing the knowledge of the prevention and treatment of common diseases, of health preservation in the different seasons, and caring more patients' needs, etc.; The theory related to health preservation should be studied and TCM hospitals or clinics should provide consultant service for healthy or sub-healthy people on disease prevention and health preservation.

3.4 Train More Elites of TCM in the Traditional Way

Many modern distinguished practitioners of TCM like Shi Jinmo 施今墨, Jiang Chunhua 姜春华, Pu Fuzhou 蒲辅周, Yue Meizhong 岳美中, Zhu Weiju 祝味菊, Deng Tietao 邓铁涛, Ren Jixue 任继学, and so and so forth, had a solid foundation of TCM, and were very creative no matter in theory or practice. Their medical attainments and skills in diagnosing and treating diseases are a wonderful integration of personal disposition, cultural accomplishments, clinical experiences, and expression of personal academic ideas. We should attach great importance to the study of these distinguished TCM experts in order to discover the way of their innovation and success both in the theoretical and clinical explorations.

More practitioners or elites of TCM should be trained in the traditional way. For example, Shandong University of TCM painstakingly chooses about 20 students every year to be trained in a more traditional way for successive 7 years: less hours in Western medicine and more hours in TCM; no hours in English and more hours in TCM classics; learn to recognize, collect, prepare, and process Chinese medicinals; learn to make different preparation forms of Chinese medicine like pill, powder, extract; learn almost all available therapies of TCM including tuina, acupuncture, moxibustion, herbal remedies; follow certain doctors or teachers to learn skills; etc.

TCM is a great treasure house of Chinese culture, and an important component part of the world civilization. Eastern culture and Western culture should be set to equal status, and both are the common spiritual wealth of the human being. As Confucius said, "Men of noble character can be harmonious but different". I do hope TCM and Western medicine can harmoniously coexist worldwide to contribute together to the human health and well-being.

Gertrude Kubiena

Applied Methodologies for Teaching, Learning, Spreading and Survival of TCM
Insights from the Beijing Workshop 2007 on Terminology

TCM teachers outside China usually simply teach TCM without reflecting methodology. In course of time they learn to give associations with familiar phenomena to overcome the cultural differences. Thus they apply the method of strangification – without being aware of this technical term. Moreover, they have to struggle with the methodologies of the underlying issues, e.g. TCM itself, correlation with Modern Western Medicine, terminology, the Chinese language and how to deal with it, translation versus interpretation, practical application, investigation (e.g. study designs) etc. The Beijing workshop 2007 with Chinese top-class experts revealed that especially terminology is not only a concern for facilitation of understanding TCM outside China. Moreover the unification of TCM terminology is taken very seriously in China as a national concern because it is considered a precondition for the survival of TCM by modernization and internationalization.

Methodology of TCM-Terminology

The problem of TCM terminology originally arises from the foreigners who want to understand Chinese Medicine. TCM terminology is a great problem for TCM students outside China: Different textbooks and teachers use different terms for one and the same matter. Therefore my original target of the Beijing workshop 2007 was the clarification of some key expressions of TCM, to facilitate TCM teaching and learning. But I learnt that standardization of TCM terminology is not only a must for foreign students; moreover it is considered essential for the survival of TCM in its motherland! Modernization and internationalization are regarded the appropriate methods to achieve this aim. Quotation Zhu Jianping: "[T]he standardization of terms of TCM became one of the keys for the modernization and internationalization of TCM"[1]. "Chinese Terms in Traditional Chinese Medicine and Pharmacy" is the title of a book published 2005 by "The National Committee for Examination and Definition of Scientific and Technological Terms". Top-class experts research since years on this topic. This shows how serious the problem is taken in China. Unfortunately the book's concept is rather adequate for Chinese scholars than for Western users: The entrances are in Chinese characters and there is no pinyin transcription. But if some issues are added the publication will help to clarify many misunderstandings about TCM in- and outside China.

Methodology of TCM Itself

Chinese Medicine submits all natural phenomena to three complex principals: Qi, yinyang, wuxing (five phases). Wallner considers these TCM basics representing a more appropriate contemporary theory of medical science than Modern Western Medicine offers (if medicine is a science at all – referring to Wallner). Nevertheless, starting to study TCM, these concepts may appear upsetting because of their complexity.

Since 36 years I am concerned with TCM and since 25 years I am teaching it. Some issues are extremely difficult to understand for TCM students. The lecture of Zhang Qicheng, a specialist for the history of TCM, clarified many problems.

We, in the West, frequently neglect the historical development of the basic theories of the TCM. The three concepts (qi, yinyang, wuxing) originate from natural, substantial phenomena, which could be experienced by the human sense organs – could be seen, heard, smelt or just felt. In this sense they were already known during the late Shang dynasty (~1700-1100 BC). In course of time they changed to metaphoric categories of Chinese philosophy, used to describe the movements of the universe. Likewise Chinese Medicine adopted these three concepts, still using them nowadays.

Nevertheless the original meaning remains implicated in their sense and this is very helpful to understand their nature. Qi, yinyang, wuxing have become models of thinking as well as philosophical categories, which are applied to explain the vital functions and the pathological

---

1 Quotation Zhu Jianping, lecture May 4th 2007

changes of the human body. All of them express a relational reality, are holistic, interrelated and show a temporal sequence. Balance and harmony are the precondition for health. Each concept is interrelated with the others and so it became usual to mention them together at one stretch. E.g. there are three main manifestations of qi: jing 精, qi 气 and shen 神. As long as we are awake jing – the most substantial stuff – is steadily transformed into qi by the qi of the middle warmer (i.e. a synonym for the digestive system). Jing rather belongs to the category yin, qi is much more yang. The third and highest manifestation shen 神 – spirit, is the most volatile / the most yang of the three qi. Shen is transformed from qi and it causes the specification of human being compared with animal's life. During sleep reversed transformation takes place; i.e. shen is transformed to qi and qi is transformed to jing.

The concept of qi

Qi originally means a sort of gas or damp, anyway a substance, like the breath, which can be seen on a cold day. The simple idea of "gas" has transformed to "the manifestation of any invisible force" (quotation Zhang Qicheng). When we refer to qi in the human body, it means a steady moving, transforming and warming, propelling and protecting substance and energy, which everything bodily and in the world is made of. Being aware of the original idea about qi as a gas-like substance, helps to understand the relation between qi 氣 and jing 精 essence – jing and as well the idea of the inseparability of material stuff and energy – an anticipation of the theories of Einstein – has its reference in these characters:

The old character for qi 氣 is a combination of the pictogram for damp 气 in the first place (the modern character for qi only uses this mutilated form) with the character for rice / grain mi 米, (standing for all sorts of nourishment). In contrast, the character for essence – jing 精 is combined from grain – mi 米 in the first place, and completed by the character for qing 青 in the second place, here used to indicate the pronunciation.

It is important to be aware that any sort of qi is made from refined substance – essence – jing 精. The quality of body-produced qi depends on the quality of the inherited constitution – represented as congenital essence – jing, and the quality of the postnatal "input" – air, food and beverages. So jing and qi are inseparable ideas: Qi 氣 is the active component of jing, 精, which has to be understood as some refined substance, created from air, food and beverages and characterized individually by the prenatal qi (derived from prenatal jing – the structive component of the inherited potential – DNA) with high potential of activity.

In Chinese Medicine, at least 15 different forms of qi can be differentiated; furthermore there are various synonyms for the specific sorts of qi, which is upsetting for the beginners in TCM:

1. Prenatal / congenital / source / essential qi – xian tian zhi qi / yuan qi / jing qi is made from prenatal jing – xian tian zhi jing. As we saw above the latter means the material basis of the inherited properties from the parents. It may be compared with the construction plan of a house or with the DNA, specifying / individualizing every substance and energy, which is formed in the course of life.
2. Postnatal / acquired qi – hou tian zhi qi is individually specified by congenital qi and made from
3. grain qi – 谷气 gu qi (food and beverages) and
4. air – 大气 da qi. These two components are the elementary basic stuff for building up all the body's substance and energy during lifetime. By the
5. 气 qi of the middle warmer – 中气 zhong qi – referring to stomach and spleen – the 谷气 gu qi – "grain qi" ist transformed to
6. 青气青气 pure qi – qing qi, which is sent from the spleen to the lung. There it mingles up with the air –大气 da qi. After positive check-up by the
7. qi of the ancestors – 宗气 zong qi it becomes
8. 真气 true qi – zhen qi. This zhen qi is divided into two parts: The very pure part becomes
9. 营气 nourishing qi – ying qi, which creates and vitalizes all body functions. According to the place, where it is acting, ying qi is called
10. 经气 channel qi – jing qi
11. 脏 服 organ qi – zang fu zhi qi
12. 正气 upright qi– zheng qi enables us to stay upright, even if we are attacked by pathogenic qi – 邪气. Defence takes place in different levels, the most superficial of which is called
13. 卫气 defence qi – wei qi, protecting the body surface from intrusion of

14. 邪气 pathogenic qi – xie qi. We are steadily exposed to potential exterior pathogens like wind, cold, dampness, dryness or summer heat. "Potential", because not everybody falls ill by exposure to these bioclimatic factors. In the first place this is a question of the relativity between the strength of xie qi and of the body's surface defence qi – wei qi. Nevertheless defence does not only occur at the surface but as well on the level of organ qi and last not least of jing qi – essential or yuan qi.
15. 浊气 Turbid qi – zhuo qi is the expression for the waste, which is expelled after descending through the intestines.

When I proudly presented this survey about qi to our Chinese colleagues Lu Guangxin, a very wise old TCM-practitioner and member of the China Academy of Chinese Medical Sciences, encountered: "Qi is simply qi!" Of course he is right, but this statement is not helpful for my students, who are confronted with all theses different sorts of qi and with all the synonyms.

The concept of yin-yang

Before lecturing about yin yang I always ask my students about their understanding of yin and yang. The most frequent answer is "contrast", as one can as well read in several reference books. The cultural and historical context is largely unknown. Zhang Qicheng pointed out that originally – in prehistoric times – yin yang referred to a shady and a sunny place. During the late Zhou dynasty (1100-256 BC) "the characters yin yang had become a philosophical category already, used to explain all the natural things and phenomena"(quotation Zhang Qicheng). Yin and yang were considered "two qi", describing freezing and unfreezing, spring thunder etc. About 500 BC (late Spring and Autumn period) yin and yang were used within the art of war – a practice, still alive in the field of wu shu, e.g. taiji quan: giving in and backward movement referring to yin, attacking and forward moving to yang. The Huangdi Neijing – the Inner Canon of the Yellow Emperor – upgraded yin yang to a metaphysical level, using it to categorize earth and heaven, female and male, water and fire etc. Furthermore in the Neijing yin and yang serve to describe relations within the human body: The body's surface is yang, the interior organs are yin, but this fact has to be seen relatively: On the surface are the superficial courses of the so called meridians or channels, which are divided into yin and yang channels: The yang channels are located where the sun may tan the skin, the yin channels at the more shady places of the body. (This example shows how important it is to be aware of the original meaning of yin and yang!) As well the interior organs are divided into yin – the zang (i.e. parenchymatous), and yang – the fu organs (i.e. hollow organs). Moreover: Many pathological changes are described as disturbance of the yin-yang-balance: If we refer to water for yin, and to fire for yang, we can easily understand the development of heat or cold within the body: Preponderance of yin causes cold, preponderance of yang heat. Like in the concept of qi we find the inseparability and interdependence of substance and function in the idea of yin and yang: if yin – substance is o.k., then function will be o.k. too. If one of the two is damaged, the other one will as well be disturbed. Still moreover we find a steady transcendence and transformation of yin and yang: There is a steady change of dark and light – night and day, ebb and tide, cold season and warm season etc.

So, talking about yin and yang we always must be aware, what are we talking about: daily life and environment or Chinese Medicine, e.g. topography, physiology or pathology. Anyway the yin yang concept is much more than a simple categorization. The yin-yang-concept implies the interrelation of substance and function, opposition and harmony, transcendence, transformation, creation and balance; to say it in a nutshell: The Yin-yang-concept describes the dynamics of the universe. In correlation with qi, there is yin qi – slowing down, calming, darkening and cooling etc. and there is yang qi – accelerating, activating and exciting, lightening and warming etc. This example is a demonstration of the inseparability of the first two of three basic TCM concepts.

The concept of wu xing – Five Phases/Five Elements

As Zhang Qicheng explains, according to actual research the Five Phases were already known as five material substances during the later Shang dynasty (1700-1100 BC). The concretization into water, wood, fire, earth and metal / gold took place during the Western Zhou dynasty (1100-770 BC), and the idea of their mutual generation was created between 770 and

476 BC (Spring and Autumn period) and worked out as well as correlated with the yin yang theory during the period of the Warring States (476-221 BC). During the Han dynasty (206 BC-220) BC) it was declared divine and – to quote Zhang Qicheng: "…wuxing became the holy unchangeable world view, methodology, and persisted until the end of the Qing dynasty" (1911).

For western people the expression "Five Elements" is upsetting, because they cannot help correlating them with the Four Elements of the Greek philosophy. Anyway the translation of the syllable "xing" is certainly not "element"! The Concise English-Chinese, Chinese-English dictionary offers the following translations: used as a verb: 1. walk, travel; 2. do, carry out; 3. be all right; used as a noun: 1. trip, 2. behaviour. Not only we westerners struggle with the translation, the Chinese do as well, because there is simply no satisfying translation, covering the sense of wu xing. Anyway "Five Phases" is better than "Five Elements, because "Phase" implicates change and movement. Zhang Qicheng quotes several attempts of sense making interpretations and correlations. E.g. already Joseph Needham struggled with the problem as there were always very contradictory ideas about how to interpret "xing".

There are on the one hand five types of basic material and on the other hand five types of basic functions. The following table coordinates materials and functions:

Material	Function
Water	Lubrication
Wood	Bending and straightening
Fire	Inflammation
Earth	Sowing and ripening
Metal/gold	Changing / following and eliminating

In former times the earth was the centre and the other four elements were arranged around it, well divided in a yin- and a yang-section (s. graphic 1).

Nowadays the Five Phases commonly are arranged in a cycle, symbolizing the mutual generation and consummation as well as the mutual restriction and rebellion against. (s. graphic 2)

Graphic 1: The Old System of the Five Phases

Originally wood, fire, metal and water were arranged around the earth in the centre. Yang is above, yin below the diagonal line. The phases which are belonging yang show a rising, those belonging to yin a sinking tendency of movement

The arrows indicate the tendency of the respective movement.
- ⇧ upward
- ⇖⇗ upward and outward
- ⇩ downward
- ⇘⇙ downward and inward

	Fire huô 火 Original yang Adolescence ⇧ South	
Wood mù 木 Yang birth ⇖⇗ East	Earth tû 土 Transformation Centre	Metal / Gold jïn 金 Old age ⇘⇙ West
	Water shuî 水 Conception Original yin ⇩ North	

Graphic 2: The Relations between the Five Phases

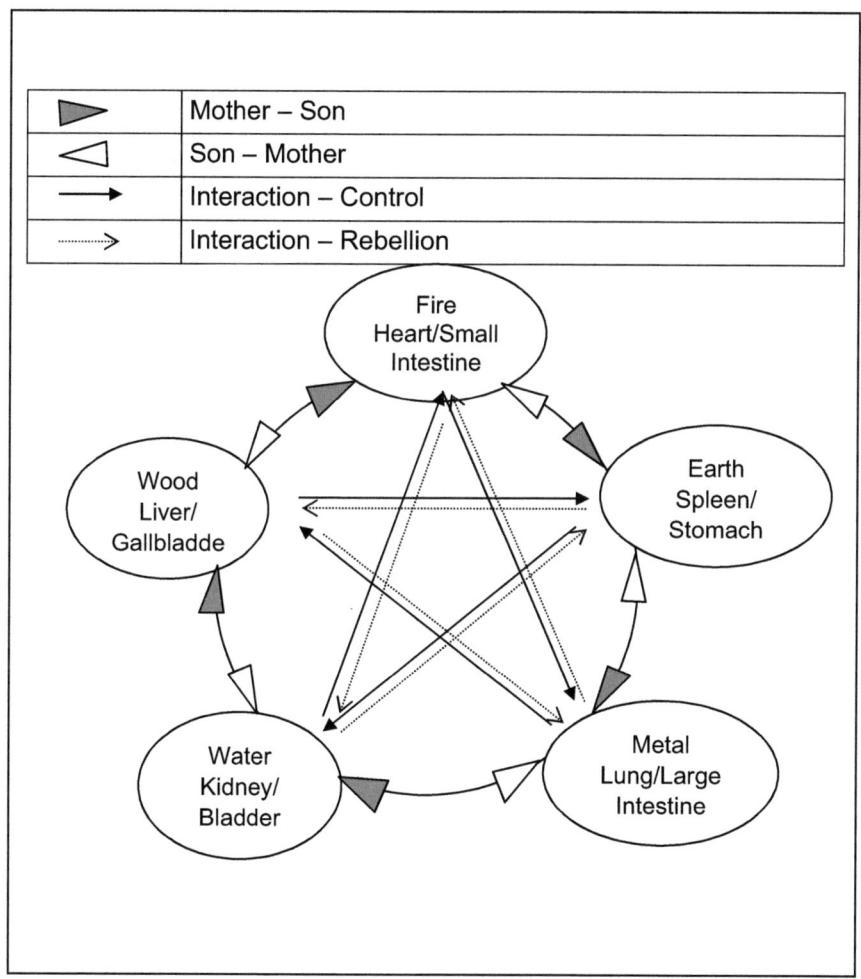

In Chinese Medicine the interior organs are correlated with the Five Phases, which serve to describe "the reality of relation and function". Any scholar of TCM uses the concept of the Five Phases to describe imbalances between the interior organs.

Anyway, the Five Phases are another example of the change from material stuff to a model of thinking.

Methodology of Correlation of TCM with Modern Western Medicine in Practice and Investigation

Western Medicine of course works with modern diagnoses and claims treatment according to "the state of the art". E.g. any gastric ulcer has to be treated in a given way. Chinese Medicine may be applied in the same way. This is called bian bing – diagnosis differentiation and it works up to a certain degree. E.g. one can buy respective remedies or for joint pain for common cold in any hotel lobby. In 1972 I was taught to apply acupuncture in the same way as Modern Western Medicine: We had to learn by heart programs for headache, abdominal pain, joint pain etc.

But the strong suite of Chinese Medicine is the pattern differentiation – bian zheng. This starts where Modern Western Medicine has its limits. Ted Kaptchuk brings a very impressive example in his famous book "The Web has no Weaver": Six patients with verified gastric ulcer were examined by TCM experts and there were six different Chinese diagnoses, requesting different treatment strategy:

Diagnosis	Treatment Strategy
1. Damp heat invading spleen	Clear damp heat from the spleen
2. Yin deficiency	Replenish yin
3. Yang deficiency	Warm and reinforce yang
4. Cold damp attacking stomach	Eliminate cold damp, warm and harmonize the stomach
5. Spleen disharmony damages liver	Harmonize spleen and liver
6. Blood stasis in stomach	Resolve blood stasis

> Mark: Modern Western Medicine treats the disease.
> Chinese Medicine treats the individual patient with his disease.

To take full advantage of this strong suite of TCM the actual modern diagnosis has to be correlated with the Chinese pattern. This is an ingenious method, holistic and unique among the medical systems of the world. In Chinese it is called bian zheng lun zhi – biàn zhèng lùn zhì 辩证论治, literally translated: identify patterns and administer treatment (of course according to the pattern!). The salient point is that the Chinese pattern directly guides to the treatment principle. E.g. if there is damp heat invading the body, one has to remove damp heat; if there is yin deficiency, one has to nourish yin; if there is yang deficiency, one has to warm and strengthen yang.

Thus one cannot simply ask for a prescription for hypertension. Only the individual Chinese diagnosis is the key to successful treatment.

The importance of thinking Chinese when treating Chinese patterns cannot be emphasized on enough: Of course, modern medicinal knowledge must not be neglected, in contrary; it has to be considered very carefully. But sometimes Chinese Medicine is simply more rapid and more effective than modern Western Medicine.

E.g. SARS: The pathogen – in the Western sense of meaning – was finally found two years after the first occurrence of SARS. Because modern Western Medicine only can treat a disease if the reason is known, it lasted a long time to find some modern treatment methods (vaccination etc). Chinese Medicine failed as well – if it was applied according to Western thinking, namely trying to stimulate the immune system with Astragalus membranaceus. But TCM was and is extremely successful – if applied according to Chinese thinking, namely considering not only the pathogen but as well the body's reaction on it, the nature of the disease, individual condition and environmental influences.

The same experience was made with several epidemics of encephalitis B. In 1956 it happened in Shijiazhuang, Hebei province. Therapy with Gypsum decoction – bai hu tang (literal white tiger soup) was very effective. 1957 the same epidemic occurred in Beijing during a very damp and warm summer. According to the successful application in Hebei, Western educated MDs also applied bai hu tang, but without positive results. Only after the famous TCM practitioner Pu Fu Zhou added Atractylodis Rhizoma – cang zhu to eliminate dampness, the therapy achieved 90 per cent rate of efficiency. 1968 in Guangdong encephalitis B was treated by the prominent physician Deng Tietao very successfully with prescriptions for summer heat with hidden dampness.[1]

All this, of course, was carried out with the respective individual and environmental adaptation. It is a pity that the result never was published in any scientific journal. In spite of the effectiveness, the evaluators – all of them MDs of Western Medicine – judged the treatment unscientific: "113 different prescriptions with 98 different herbs – that is not a uniform concept and so we cannot accept it."[2]

This individuality complicates clinical investigations on TCM in the modern sense. The ideal modern study design excludes as many items as possible. The result of the application of this technique has shown up with the recent German multicenter acupuncture study: Thousands of head- or low-backache patients received either correct or sham acupuncture and the result was compared with conventional drug therapy. The therapeutic scheme was given. The result showed superiority of as well sham as well correct acupuncture over the conventional drug therapy. There was no statistically significant difference between correct and sham acupuncture.

Methodology of the Chinese Language and How to Deal with

Chinese is a beautiful melodious language, but unfortunately often violated by foreigners. Bob Flaws claims any TCM student to study Chinese first. I think, this carries things too far, but some basic knowledge of the Chinese language is indispensable.

Chinese is a polysyllabic language with monosylabic infrastructure. That means: 1 syllable = 1 character = 1 word = autosemantica. Classical Chinese uses exclusively autosemantica. In modern Chinese there are 40% autosemantica, the rest are synsemantica (i.e. consisting of more than one syllable). If a term consists of two syllables, frequently every part has the same meaning on its own. E.g. 孩子 hai zi means child, but only 孩 hai or only 子 zi as well means child.

---

1 Wang Xin-Yuan / Pu Gong-Ying: Lemology in Traditional Chinese Medicine: With Prevention and Treatment of SARS as A Case in Point.
2 Lin Zhongpeng, personal information

Compared with English, which has 8000 syllables, Chinese has very few, namely 411, which are differentiated by the four tones into 1338. Therefore one syllable has different meanings, even with one and the same tone. E.g. for jing with the first tone there are more than 15 different characters. Therefore the question "What does jing mean?" can only be answered by looking up the Chinese character and from the context.

Let us look at the translations of the Chinese character 经 jing in the Concise Chinese-English English-Chinese Dictionary: Used as noun: 1. warp (of textile); 2. longitude; 3. scripture, classics. Used as verb: 1. pass through, undergo; 2. manage, deal in; 3. stand, endure. Moreover in Chinese Medicine this character as well stands for the acupuncture channels and for menstruation.

A group of German TCM experts emphasizes on mainly using Latin. Quite a reasonable attempt because Latin is more than international, namely supranational. However they mix up Latin with Chinese, moreover in Wade Giles transcription. So unsurprisingly internationalization of this system did not occur. Unfortunately several Western TCM teachers preferably use Chinese in their lectures. Some even insist on exclusively using it. And – one can't help the impression: The worse their Chinese the more they use it. This fact creates a great problem, when Western and Chinese teachers alternating give lectures: The students have in mind the mutilated pronunciation of the Western teacher and don't understand the correct pronunciation of the Chinese teacher!

Inevitably the question arises: Why should Western teachers use Chinese at all in TCM lectures? The answer: Because several basic ideas of TCM cannot be translated in a satisfactory manner; e.g. qi, yinyang, wuxing. Anyway, even if not every TCM student or even teacher can study the Chinese language extensively, some very basic principles should be made clear from the beginning; furthermore some rules of pronunciation should be given.

Methodology of TCM translation

The language of the classics is different to modern Chinese. Therefore the Chinese classics are not simply understandable by any literate Chinese!

To say it in a nutshell: There are two possibilities for translation: literal and interpretational.[1]

1. literal

Quoting Peter Newman: There are four advantages of literal translation:
   a) Correct
   b) Concentrated
   c) Systematic
   d) Re-translation English-Chinese only from literal translation possible

The following example may serve to illustrate the advantages of literal translation: 风火眼 feng huo yan – literally wind fire eye – stands for a certain form of conjunctivitis, caused by exterior wind-hea, e.g. hey fevert. But there are different sorts of conjunctivitis by different pathomechanisms! Not any conjunctivitis is wind fire eye! So if one re-translates any type of conjunctivitis into Chinese as feng huo yan the result will be the full catastrophe!

2. interpretational

Zhang Qicheng presents an interesting example, illustrating the problem of literal translation without connotations. The background: While in China each acupuncture point has its individual name, in the West a system of point-numbering, following the course of the channel, is usual. The Western system is not unintelligent: The numbers of the points follow the course of the channel. When I went to China for the first time – 1986 – this caused certain problems: Our Chinese teachers were not familiar with our system of point numbering, and we were not familiar with the Chinese acupuncture point names. Meanwhile most of the Chinese teachers have adapted to the Western numbering system. In my opinion neglecting the proper acupuncture point names is a pity! These can tell us a lot about the specific properties of a point – but only with known context! Zhang Qichengs example: "'gongsun' (the name of an acumoxa point) has been translated as 'grandfather and grandson'". Of course this does not say anything about the specific properties of the point. In "Acupuncture, Meridian Theory and Acupuncture Points" Li Ding writes: "'Gong' was originally a respectful form of address for high officials. 'Sun' means grandson. ...The point is the connecting point of the meridian, from which a branch emerges,

---

1 Lecture Lan Fengli, April 28th 2007

hence the name ´gong sun´ (grandson of a prince)". Quite a good explanation, but still it lacks the very specific property of this point, which is called Spleen 4 in Western terminology; because every channel has a luo connecting point!

But if one knows that "sun" here has to be seen with another background than simply "grandson", the matter clarifies: Namely, this point is the luo connecting point of the very tiny collaterals, the capillaries, which are called sun luo, because they are the twigs of the twigs of the twigs. If we now interpret with "prince" or "official of the sun luo" its specific property becomes obvious. So I think, simplification is legitimate, e.g. for acupuncture; but the proper names with the appropriate connotations are essential for the understanding.

Methodology of Practical Application, e.g. Prescriptions

In China of course prescriptions are written down in Chinese characters, excluding any misunderstanding. When this practice – in pin yin transcription – is adopted outside China, it may lead to lethal misunderstandings, e.g. the scandal in Belgium: Stephania root – han fang ji was prescribed, but the patients received Aristolochia root – guang fang ji. The follows: In more than 200 cases cancer of the kidney, damage, dead and accusations. How could this happen? Because both of the drugs may be called simply fang ji! If the prescription contains the Latin name, the pharmacist has to follow it. Up to now I don't know if the pharmacists got the wrong stuff from the dealer – Aristolochia instead of Stephania, or if the prescribers missed to make a correct prescription in pinyin and in Latin.

Conclusion: Outside China it is obligatory to use Latin in the first place and pin yin in the second one.

Methodology of TCM-Teaching

Because of the cultural differences the approach is different in China and in the West. In China TCM studying usually starts with lecture of the classic textbooks. My Chinese friends say "it is boring in the beginning". But Chinese students are used to accept what the teacher teaches, without many questioning. And so they start to learn by heart things, which they can not yet understand. Practical application of the stuff finally brings understanding.

In the West one cannot start like this, students are more critical and want a plausible explanation for everything. Because human memory always clings to associations, we learnt from Wallner, that, what we are doing is called strangification. I.e. we use allegories from familiar phenomena to transport complex issues of TCM. A rule of my own, which I learned from Harry Lorayne[1]: The more drastic the better. Another stupefying experience: Chinese teachers use this method as well! [2]

Summary

TCM teachers out side and even inside China commonly use the method of strangification without being aware of doing so. The target is to facilitate teaching and learning the complex stuff and to overcome the cultural difference. The latter not only exists between China and the West but as well between the generators of the basic theory of science of TCM and the nowadays Chinese students. My recommendation for teaching TCM outside China: Don't emphasize too much on the cultural difference, better transport the absolute logical drive of the TCM basics.

Dealing with the methodology of teaching TCM involuntary leads to dealing as well with the methodologies of the underlying issues:

The methodology of TCM proper: All natural phenomena are submitted to three complex principals: Qi, Yin-Yang and Five Phases. These three theories are widely interrelated and have many common issues: They changed from natural phenomena, perceptible with the sense organs to untranslatable models of thinking, implying substance and function, relativity, transformation, change and temporal sequence. The historical development has to be emphasized on more.

Concerning the methodology of the use of the Chinese language in teaching or discussing TCM: Because the basic ideas if TCM actually are not translatable, the use of some Chinese expressions is inevitable. It is not possible for every foreign TCM teacher to learn the Chinese language absolutely correct. But TCM teachers have to know and to teach at least

---

1 Lorayne H (1957) How to Develop a Super-Power Memory
2 Beijing Workshop 2007, Lecture Jiang Wenyue, April 30th 2007

its structure (polysyllabic language with monosyllabic structure) and the fact that the language changed from the creating-time of the classics to nowadays. And whoever is concerned with TCM has to have at least an idea about its pronunciation.

Translation: From the two possibilities – literal or interpretational – none is fully satisfying. I vote for literal translation with connotations.

Correlation of TCM and Modern Western Medicine: The right methodology of approaching a modern Western diagnosis is to point out which Chinese pattern it is fitting. The name of the Chinese pattern describes what is happening within the body and guides directly to the right treatment. Modern Western Medicine starts where TCM has its limits, e.g. operations, antibiotics, intensive care etc. On the other hand TCM is superior where Modern Western Medicine has its limits, i.e. still unknown or untreatable diseases in Western Medicine. TCM´s worldwide unique method of directly correlating Chinese pattern diagnosis and therapeutic principal – bian zheng lun zhi – selection of therapy based on the preceding Chinese pattern differentiation – characterizes once more TCM as holistic.

Practical application of and investigation on TCM: Western methodology leads to bad results in both cases. E.g. SARS and Encephalitis B can be treated very well with Chinese Medicine, but only if Chinese thinking is applied. Western thinking in using Chinese remedies inevitably causes a flop.

Clinical trials as well usually end in a flop if they are carried out following the very restrictive usual modern study designs. Chinese Medicine includes individual and environmental parameters, which are usually neglected by the Modern Western Medicine.

The complex terminology of TCM is not only a problem for foreign students. Moreover the standardization of terminology is considered the key for survival of TCM in its motherland via modernization and internationalization.

References

Beijing Fremdspracheninstitut, Abteilung für Deutsch: Neues Chinesisch - Deutsches Wörterbuch. Beijing waiguoyu xueyuan deyu xi: "Xin Han-De Cidian". Shangwu yinshuguan chuban. Shangwu yin Verlag, Beijing, Erstauflage August 1985. 北京 外国语 学 院德语系 . 新 汉德 词典 . 编 写组 编。商务印书馆出版. ISBN: 7-100-00096-3/H 40

Beijing Workshop 2007: "Comparative Analysis of Central Expressions of Traditional Chinese Medicine (TCM) in the Context of Modern Western Medicine". April 23rd – May 9th 2007, Beijing, Swissotel. Personal information

Flaws B. (1994) Statements of Fact in Traditional Chinese Medicine. Blue Poppy Press, Inc. Boulder. ISBN:0-936185-52-x

Li Ding (1991) Acupuncture, Meridian Theory and Acupuncture Points. Foreign Language Press, Beijing. ISBN: 0-8351-2221-2 and 7-119-00405-0

Lorayne H. (1985, First Printing 1974) How to develop a super-power memory. A Signet Book, New American Library, a division of Penguin books USA Inc., 1633 Broadway, New York ISBN: 0-451-16036-3

Manser Martin H (chief editor) (2004) Concise English-Chinese / Chinese-English Dictionary (Third Edition). The Commercial Press & Oxford University Press. ISBN: 978-7-100-03933-8 / ISBN-10: 7-100-03933-9

National committee for examination und definition of scientific und technological terms: see quan guo kexue jishu mingci shending weiyuanhui /

Quanguo kexue jishu mingci shending weiyuanhui: National committee for examination und definition of scientific und technological terms: Chinese terms in Traditional Chinese Medicine und Pharmacy. 2004, kexue chubanshe, Beijing. ISBN: 7030151542

Wallner F.G (2001) http://www.univie.ac.at/constructive-realism/

Wallner, F. G (2005) Structure and Relativity. Verlag Peter Lang, Frankfurt. ISBN : 978-3-631-51865-

Wiseman N. (1995) English-Chinese Chinese-English Dictionary of Chinese Medicine. Hunan Kexue Jishu Chubanshe, Changsha ISBN: 7-5357-1656-3/H

Lan Fengli

Metaphor, *Qu Xiang Bi Lei* and Chinese Medicine

The thesis explains metaphor, the thinking way of *qu xiang bi lei*, and their philosophical foundations, takes some examples to illustrate how metaphors are used to state and construct the theoretical system of Chinese medicine and to develop Chinese medicine in both theoretical and practical explorations in the thinking way of *qu xiang bi lei,* and finally draws a conclusion that metaphor in the thinking way of *qu xiang bi lei* is an important means and process of stating, constructing and developing Chinese medicine.

Introduction

Modernization of Chinese medicine must be directed by scientific methodology, and scientific methodology belongs in the field of philosophy, esp. the field of philosophy of science. The key tone of the modern Western philosophy focuses on language analysis and understanding. Today, language is redefined as the means and process of human beings cognizing, understanding and stating the world.[1] The founding of philosophy of language at the beginning of the last century is another "Copernican revolution" in the history of philosophy,[2] which has deeply influenced philosophy of science, highlighting the vital role of linguistic analysis in the scientific methodology, thus promoting the development of modern logic.

Modern logic stresses the role of language, regards a scientific theory as a language system, being composed of word items, sentences, and their logic relationships. When analyzing Chinese medical system, how the basic Chinese medical concepts and theories were formed, stated

---

1 Pan Wenguo. Redefining Language: Means and Process of Human Being Cognizing and Stating the Genuine World[J]. (Hongkong) Chinese Philology Correspondence. 2002, 2.
2 Xu Youyu. "Copernican" Revolution: Linguistic Transfer in Philosophy[M]. Shanghai: Joint Publishing House, 1994: 1.

and constructed, and how Chinese medicine has been developed should be clarified in the first place for the purpose of understanding the system itself, bridging traditional Chinese medicine and modern Western medicine in deep level and complementing each other, thus laying foundation for modernization of Chinese medicine.

1. Metaphor, *Qu Xiang Bi Lei*, and Their Philosophical Foundations

1.1 Metaphor

Metaphor is an important field of study shared in rhetoric, linguistics and philosophy. Metaphor originally refers to a rhetorical skill, a figure of speech, but is given a much more extensive meaning by logic pragmatics, referring to phenomena of meaning transfer of language in the course of expression and exchange.[1] As a process of semantic constitution, metaphor fulfills this process by means of "deviation". This deviation is a result of diversion of human beings' intention. The motivation of semantic constitution comes from human beings' cognitive abilities contained in metaphor.

Metaphor is also a basic cognitive activity. Metaphor in language use is the medium as well as the result of metaphoric cognitive activities of human beings. Metaphor is an indispensable means by which human beings cognize the world.

Language by itself contains a system of metaphor. This system is closely connected with human beings' thinking system. Languages and symbols have become a complete model that a nation regards the world. Human beings have made themselves a whole. While metaphor is used, it brings back to life the image of human beings in nature and the nature of human beings as well.[2]

1.2 Qu Xiang Bi Lei

The *Origin of Chinese Characters* (shuo wen jie zi, 《说文解字》) states that "xiang, with long nose and teeth, is a big mammal in the Southern Yue area", so the original meaning of "xiang" is elephant. In remote antiquity,

---

1 Zhou Liquan. Logic: Theory of Correct Thinking and Efficient Communication[M]. Beijing: People's Publishing House, 1994: 489.
2 Gao Liping. Philosophying Metaphor[J]. Journal of Shandong TV University, 2006, 2.

the elephant had lived in the Central Plains of China. Later on, the elephant had to migrate south because of the changes in climate, so the people in the Central Plains had few opportunity to see elephant again. Han Fei-Zi (韩非子), a famous philosopher and the representative of the Legalists of the late Warring States Period (475-221B.C.), said in his *Jie Lao Pian* (《解老篇》) that "people seldom see the live elephant, but has gained the skeleton of a dead one, so they can imagine what it is like after investigating the picture or image of its skeleton. Therefore, all in people's imagination is known as 'xiang'". This quotation also reveals the mystery of the origin of the Chinese compound "xiang xiang" (想象, literally "thinking or imagining elephant", means imagination), setting off "xiang 象"'s "imagining" cultural connotations.

Based on the direct experiences the ancient obtained from observing objects, *qu xiang*, literally means "taking or selecting images", refers to a thinking way of applying concrete images of the objective world and its symbols to express and think in the way of metaphorizing, symbolizing, associating, and analogizing, thus reflecting universal relationships and rules of the things or objects.[1] *Bi lei*, or analogizing, is a thinking process, which compares, finds, and catches the similarities between the two different kinds of things, then migrate or move and infer the knowledge of one thing to the other by applying metaphor on the basis of observing object or phenomenon and taking image.

Qu xiang bi lei can be summarized into four steps or links as stated in *the Book of Changes*: 1) Observing object or phenomenon (*guan wu* 观物): directly observing object or phenomenon; 2)Taking image (*qu xiang* 取象): summarizing and refining the image of the object or phenomenon after repeatedly observing and feeling it; 3)Analogizing (*bi lei* 比类): comparing the things which need to know with the "image (*xiang* 象)"; 4) Understanding the Way or Rule (*ti dao* 体道): finding the rules, which can be achieved by applying metaphor.

Metaphors in the thinking way of qu xiang bi lei, the core methodology of Chinese medicine, play a vital role in stating, constructing and developing the theoretical system and clinical practice of Chinese medicine mainly in the following three aspects: 1) naming basic concepts, stating

---

1 Xing Yu-Rui. The Theories and Methodology in the *Huang Di's Inner Classic*. Xi'an: Shaanxi Science and Technology Press, 2004: 189.

and constructing the theoretical system; 2) grasping the hidden essence or telling the interior through observing the external image or manifestation; and 3) inferring the unknown through the known image.

1.3 Philosophical Foundations of Metaphor and *Qu-Xiang Bi Lei*

The theme of Chinese philosophy is to probe into the relationship between "the heaven and human being", or the relationship between "the Way of heaven and the Way of human being", regarding the heaven as human being's heaven and the human being as heaven's human being. Therefore, the heaven and the human being unite each other, and correspond to each other.

The theoretical system of Chinese medicine has formed on the idea of "the heaven and the human being uniting and corresponding to each other". *Huang Di's Inner Classic ·Plain Questions· Discourse on Protecting Life and Preserving Physical Appearance* (huang di nei jing su wen· bao ming quan xing lun, 《黄帝内经素问·宝命全形论》) states that "Man is born on the earth, hanging his life to the heaven. The union of qi of the heaven and earth gives birth to Man. Man can adapt himself to the seasons for the Heaven and Earth are his parents". That is to say, man or human being is the outcome of the evolution of the heaven, the earth and the nature to a certain period; and the human being and the heaven share the common constituent: qi. *The Book of Changes* states that "the beings with the similar or same sound correspond to each other, and the beings being composed of the same constituent–qi attract each other". Therefore, the same constituent (qi) is the very basis of "the heaven and the human being uniting and corresponding to each other".

The worldview determines the methodology. Chinese medicine believes that everything in the world is universally related to each other, that the world is composed of the same constituent, and that the immense variety of things and phenomena in the world share some same characteristics at different levels, different categories, and different aspects, and moreover, there exist many necessary relationships among them. Actually, these viewpoints are the philosophical foundation of metaphor and the thinking way of *qu xiang bi lei*.

Languages are metaphoric in its essence and nature. We should not content ourselves to the present state of language. We have to trace back to the origins of words if we want to discover the ties which link the words and their references.[1] (translated from Chinese translation)

Chinese characters are ideographic writing (as opposed to phonetic writing), and *qu xiang bi lei*, is the core thinking way of Chinese medicine, therefore, metaphor is universal in Chinese medical language from words, phrases to sentences, reflecting how basic Chinese medical concepts and theories were formed, stated, and constructed, and how Chinese medicine has been developed, determining that Chinese medicine is a metaphor system. Therefore, the metaphor system formed on the basis of the thinking way of *qu xiang bi lei* is the deep structure of Chinese medicine.

2. Metaphor: Stating and Constructing the Theoretical System of Chinese Medicine in the Thinking Way of *Qu Xiang Bi Lei*[2]

Metaphor is a means and process of stating and constructing the theoretical system of Chinese medicine in the way of *qu xiang bi lei*. Qi, yin-yang, the five phases (wood, fire, earth, metal, and water), *jing luo*, and *zang fu*, the fundamental concepts and theories of Chinese medicine, were all formed by means of metaphors in the way of observing phenomena, taking images, and then reasoning from analogy. That is to say, the related images, functional models, and theories of qi, yin-yang, five phases, *jing luo,* and *zang fu*, are stated and constructed through the process of observing phenomena, cognizing their images, esp. their functional, dynamic images, and then reasoning from analogy, finally forming these specific concepts and theories in Chinese medicine.

2.1 Qi

The concept and theory of "qi" in Chinese medicine were gradually formed by means of metaphor in the way of observing and taking the image of air or vapor in the nature and analogizing.

---

1 Translator Gan Yang, Author Ernst Cassirer. An Essay on Man [M]. Shanghai: Shanghai Translation Publishing House, 2004: 152, 158. (Original Version: An Essay on Man: An Introduction to a Philosophy of Human Culture, New Heaven: Yale University Press, 1944)
2 Lan Fengli. A Corpus-Based Study on English Translation of the Basic Concepts in Ancient Chinese Medical Texts. Postdoctoral Dissertation. Shanghai: Shanghai Jiaotong University, April, 2008: 60-111.

The Origin of Chinese Characters • Qi Part (shuo wen jie zi •qi bu, 《说文解字•气部》) states that *"Qi* refers to thin, floating clouds. The character 气 is a pictographic character." The character 气 in *Jia Gu Wen*, the inscriptions on bones or tortoise shells of the Shang Dynasty (c. 16th-11th century B.C.), was written as "川", which resembles air current, evaporating and rising, whose image is just like cloud, will disappear very soon and become invisible. Therefore, qi is invisible and formless, exists everywhere, can be gathered into a form, for instance, *qi* can be condensed into water. *Qi* at this moment actually referred to air or vapor.

Soon afterwards, the *qi* which surrounds and congests the space of the human beings was abstracted into the *qi* which bears a material meaning in philosophical sense. Philosophers of materialism of the Spring Autumn and Warring States Period (770-221B.C.) believed that qi is the basic material constituting the world, and that everything in the universe comes into being by the movement and mutation of qi. For example, *Book of Changes • Section Xi Ci,* (zhou yi •xi ci, 《周易•系辞》) , states that "everything is transformed and generated by the enshrouding [qi] of the heaven and earth".

Later on, ancient Chinese medical experts introduced "*qi*" into the medical field at the right moment. And then, "*qi*" became a medium or bridge between the natural philosophy of the pre-Qin days (i.e. before 221 B.C. when the First Emperor of Qin united China) and Chinese medicine. The concept and theory of "*qi*" gradually formed in TCM.

In the time of Huangdi's Inner Classic, "qi" is regarded not only as the basic material constituting the world, but also as the basic material constituting the human being which can be transformed into blood, essence, and body fluid, etc., and the normal functional activities of the life which is governed by "qi" is known as Shen or spirit. For example, *Huangdi's Inner Classic·Plain Questions • Discourse on Protecting Life and Preserving Physical Appearance* (huang di nei jing su wen • baoming quanxing lun, 《黄帝内经素问•宝命全形论》) states that "The human being is generated by qi of the heaven and earth, and is completed by the law of the four seasons"; And that "the union of *qi* of the heaven and earth gives birth to the human being". Actually, there are abundant accounts of *qi* in the *Plain Questions*. Only the monosyllabic word "*qi*" appears 1176 times in *Plain Questions*. Almost all the 79 existing chapters of the *Plain Questions* discuss *qi*. All the theories and skills of the *Plain Questions* are related to *qi*.

And there are various *qi* with a multitude of names in the *Plain Questions*, such as yin *qi*, yang *qi*; clear *qi*, turbid *qi*; heaven *qi*, earth *qi*; right *qi* or healthy *qi*, evil *qi* or pathogenic *qi*; nutritive *qi*, defensive *qi*; seasonal *qi*, visceral *qi*, meridian *qi*; and so and so forth.[1]

According to *A Concise Dictionary of Chinese Medicine* (jian ming zhong yi ci dian,《简明中医词典》), *qi* in TCM bears the following meanings: ① nutritious, essential substance flowing inside the body, such as food qi, breathed air. ② functional activities of the *zang-fu* organs in a general sense, such as visceral *qi* (i.e, the functional activities of the *zang-fu* organs); *qi* can also be classified into original *qi*, nutritive *qi*, defensive *qi*, *pectoral* qi, etc. according to its source, distribution, and function. ③ the location or stage of pattern identification of warm diseases.[2]

2.2 Yin-Yang

The concept and theory of "yin-yang" in Chinese medicine were gradually formed by means of metaphor in the way of observing and taking the image of directions of a mountain or a river in the nature and analogizing.
Yin originally refers to the northern side of a mountain or the southern side of a river. *Han Fei Zi· Shuo Lin Shang* (《韩非子·说林上》) states that "夏居山之阴", which means "Xia lives at the northern side of a mountain". *Lie Zi · Tang Wen* (《列子·汤问》) states that "达于汉阴", which means "Arrive at the southern side of Han(shui) River". Yang originally refers to the southern side of a mountain or the northern side of a river. *Book of Documents ·Yugong* (shang shu ·yu gong,《尚书·禹贡》) states that "岷山之阳，至于衡山", which means "from the southern side of Minshan mountain to Hengshan Mountain". *Book of Songs· Qin's Tone ·Weiyang* (shi jing·qin feng·wei yang,《诗经·秦风·渭阳》) states that "我送舅氏，日至渭阳", which means "I see my uncle, to the northern side of Wei(shui) River in the daytime". Then, the original meanings of yin-yang are summarized as "the side facing the sun being yang and the reverse side being yin".

---

1 Lan Fengli. The Influence of *Huang Di's Inner Classic* on *The Origin of Chinese Characters*[J], Chinese Journal of Medical History, 2006, 36(4): 201-205.
2 Li Jingwei, Qu Yongxin, Yu Ying'ao, et al. A Concise Dictionary of Chinese Medicine. Beijing: China Press of Traditional Chinese Medicine, 2001: 173.

2.2.1 Exploring the Origin of Yin-Yang in Chinese Medicine

It was Bo Yang Fu 伯阳父 of the last years of Western Zhou Dynasty (C. 1100-771B.C.) that first used the word yin-yang, gave it the abstract meaning of opposition, and used it to explain natural phenomena. He believed that "yang hides [inside] and can not come out, yin is forced and can not ascend, and then earthquake ensues" (*Guo Yu •Zhou Yu,* 《国语•周语》). Fan Li 范蠡 of the last years of Spring-Autumn Period (770-476B.C.) said that "yang in its extreme becomes yin, and yin in its extreme becomes yang; the sun in the end rises again, and the moon in the full wanes" (*Guo Yu •Yue Yu,* 《国语• 越语》), which was the first and earliest formulation of waxing-waning and transformation of yin-yang. *Lao Zi • 42nd Chapter* (《老子•四十二章》) states that "everything in the universe bears yin and embraces yang, where the central and harmonious qi makes them in harmony". This quotation affirms that the contradictory qualities of yin-yang are intrinsic attributes of everything.

Book of Changes (yi zhuan, 《易传》) further advances that "one yin and one yang makes Tao", which abstracts yin-yang to the extensive universality and regards yin-yang as the fundamental rule of the universe for the first time. *Book of Changes* also uses yin-yang to make a comparison of social phenomena, and yin-yang has by extension come to imply the relationship between upward and downward, monarch and ministers, wife and husband, etc. Joseph Needham believed that yin-yang as definite philosophical term appears in the *Book of Changes.* Dong Zhongshu's *Chun Qiu Fan Lu* (董仲舒《春秋繁露》) states that "the heaven has yin-yang, the human being also has yin-yang. Yin qi of the heaven rises and yin qi of the human being will respond it to rise, while yin qi of the human being rises and yin qi of the heaven will respond it to rise too. The principles or ways are the same".

Chinese medicine inherits and develops the idea of yin-yang in the *Book of Changes.* Not all of the yin-yang in ancient medical texts is abstract in philosophical sense. For example, among the medical books unearthed in the *Mawangdui* Han Tomb 马王堆汉墓出土医书, *Ten Questions* (shi wen 《十问》) discusses the way of meeting yin [the female's genitals]; *Methods of Integrating Yin and Yang* (he yin-yang fang 《合阴阳方》) on the methods of copulation of the male and female; *Supreme Way of the Land under Heaven* (tian xia zhi dao tan 《天下至道谈》) on harms and benefits of sexual intercourse; *Way of Preserving Health* (yang sheng fang

《养生方》) and *Miscellaneous Therapies* (za liao fang 《杂疗方》) on function of sexual intercourse and antenatal instruction.

The theory of yin-yang is easy to tally with the male and female in the sexual intercourse. So, it is very natural to use the principles of yin-yang to explain the sexual intercourse or even use yin-yang as a synonym or euphemism of the sexual intercourse in the above-mentioned works. These works on sexual intercourse press close to the philosophy of yin-yang on one end and to the medical life on the other. So yin-yang can be regarded as a bridge between philosophy and medicine. Thus, it is very common in ancient Chinese medical texts to adopt yin-yang to represent male and female and sexual intercourse as stated in the *Mawangdui* medical books. Moreover, ancient Chinese medical classics have applied yin-yang theory extensively into the medical field in accordance with thinking way of *qu xing bi lei*, or taking images and analogizing. For example, yin-yang in concrete medical texts may refer to some specific medical meanings, such as the male and female, sex or sexual activity, yin-yang meridians, yin-yang pathogens, yin-yang *qi*, *cun* pulse and *chi* pulse, etc.

In the *Book of Changes*, yin-yang is mainly used in the field of natural philosophy; while in TCM, yin-yang is used not only in philosophical field, but also in medical field, and yin-yang is an ingenious unification of philosophical and medical senses. *Huangdi's inner Classic* (huang di nei jing, 《黄帝内经》) makes a more systematic and definite expression on the ideas of interdependence, waning-waxing, transformation, harmony of yin-yang implied in the *Book of Changes*, develops these ideas in combination with medical practice, and makes yin-yang theory become the guiding theory of TCM.

2.2.2 Understanding Yin-Yang in the Thinking Way of Qu Xiang Bi Lei

As a pair of philosophical concepts, yin-yang in essence is to summarize the dynamic images of things or phenomena. Generally speaking, things that are mobile, external, upward, ascending, warm, hot, bright, hyperactive, or pertaining to functional activities can be classified as *Yang*; those that are unmoving, internal, downward, descending, cold, dull, hypoactive, or pertaining to materials (or structures) can be classified as *Yin*. (See table 1)

Table 1 Examples of *Yin-Yang*

YIN	YANG
the earth	the sky
the moon	the sun
water	Fire
night	day
cloudy	clear
dark (dull)	bright
cold (cool)	heat (warm)
heavy	light
still	move
internal	external
downward	upward
hypoactive	hyperactive
structure (material)	function
negative	positive
descending	ascending
female	male
death	life
abdomen	back
blood	qi
Five zang organs	Six fu organs

Based on the different characteristics of the images of *Yin* and *Yang*, all things in the universe can be classified as one or the other in accordance with the thinking way of *qu xiang bi lei*. The attribute of yin or yang has nothing to do with concrete materials or shapes, and is only determined by their dynamic functions, actions and relationships instead. For example, water pertains to yin for the image of water being cool, moistening and flowing downwards corresponds to yin; fire to yang for the image of fire being warming and rising corresponds to yang. Heaven pertains to yang for the image of celestial qi being light, lucid, ascending and floating corresponds to yang; earth to yin for the image of terrestrial qi being heavy, turbid, descending and sinking corresponds to yin.

Similarly, Chinese medicine often regards *qi*, which has a propelling and warming function, as Yang; blood, which has a nourishing and moistening function, as Yin. The organic structure, the physiological functional activities of the body, as well as the signs and symptoms of pathological changes, can all be differentiated on the basis of the characteristics of the images of *Yin* and *Yang*. (see Table 2)

Table 2 Pattern Identification According to Yin and Yang

Yang Pattern	*Yin* Pattern
1. Fever, perspiration, hyperfunction	Chills or aversion to cold, hypofunction
2. Raised basal metabolic rate	Reduced basal metabolic rate
3. High temperature	Low temperature
4. Profuse perspiration	Reduced perspiration
5. Raised systolic blood pressure	Low systolic blood pressure
6. Raised diastolic blood pressure	Low diastolic blood pressure
7. Increased gastric peristalsis	Reduced gastric peristalsis
8. Sympathetic hyperactivity	Parasympathetic hyperactivity
9. Intolerance of heat	Intolerance of cold
10. Red or rosy complexion	Pale complexion
11. Desire for cold drink and food	Desire for hot drink and food
12. Dry tongue, with thirst	Moistened tongue, without thirst
13. Yellow urine	Clear urine
14. Normal quantity of saliva, normal salivation	Much saliva, hyper-salivation
15. Constipation	Diarrhea

Therefore, in short, the meaning of *Yin-Yang* is extremely simple, yet very profound. One can seemingly understand it on a rational level, and yet, continually find new connotations or expressions of it in the theoretical system and clinical practice of Chinese medicine, and, indeed, in life as well for the concept and theory of yin-yang has formed and will continually gain its new connotations in accordance with the thinking way of *qu xiang bi lei*, as stated in the *Huangdi's Inner Classic·Plain Questions· Great Discourse on Images Corresponding to Yin-Yang* (huang di nei jing su wen • yin-yang ying xiang da lun, 《黄帝内经素问•阴阳应象大论》) states that

Yin and yang, they are
the Way of heaven and earth,
the fundamental principles [governing] the myriad beings,
father and mother to all changes and transformations,
the basis and beginning of generating and killing,
the palace of spirit brilliance.[1]

2.3 Five Phases: Wood, Fire, Soil, Metal, and Water

In actual fact, the concept and theory of five phases was put forward earlier than that of qi and yin-yang as first stated in the *Book of Documents. The Fundamental Principles* (shang shu· hong fan, 《尚书·洪范》), which comes from observing and taking the images of the five objects: wood, fire, soil, metal and water in the nature, and analogizing.

The concept of five phases in classical Chinese philosophy evolved from the ancient concepts: "five directions" and "five materials". According to the records of oracle inscriptions of the Yin-Shang Dynasty (殷商 c. 16th-11th century B.C.) on the tortoise shells or animal bones, the Yin people (殷人) termed the Shang's territory "Center Shang", being juxtaposed to "East Land", "South Land", "West land", and "North Land". Thereby, the whole territory was divided into five parts, and then the concept of "five directions" formed.

In the late period of Western Zhou Dynasty and Spring-Autumn period (C. 1100-476 B.C.), theory of "the five directions" was followed by the theory of "the five materials". Shi Bo 史伯 of the late period of Western Zhou Dynasty said that "the metal, wood, water, fire and soil are mixed to generate one hundred items" (*Guo Yu ·Zhen Yu,* 《国语·郑语》) . Zi Han 子罕 of the Spring-Autumn period said that "the heaven gives birth to the five materials. People use them together. Either can not be disposed with" (*Zuo Zhuan,* 《左传·襄公二十七年》) .

The writing record of generalization of the concrete material concept "five materials" to the philosophical concept "five phases" starts with *Book of Documents. The Fundamental Principles* (shang shu· hong fan, 《尚书·洪范》), which states that "the five phases: the first is water, the second is

---

1 Unschuld, Paul U. HUANG DI NEI JING SU WEN: Nature, Knowledge, Imagery in An Ancient Chinese Medical Text[M]. Berkeley, Los Angeles and London: University of California Press, 2003: 86.

fire, the third is wood, the fourth is metal, the fifth is soil. Water is moistening and downward flowing. Fire is flaming upward. Wood is bending and straightening. Metal is transforming and changing. Soil, then, is sowing and reaping. Moistening and downward flowing generates salty [flavor]. Flaming upward generates bitter [flavor]. Bending and straightening generates sour [flavor]. Transforming and changing generates acrid [flavor]. Sowing and reaping generates sweet [flavor]". It is thus clear that the five phases do not refer to the concrete five materials any more, but to five kinds of functional attributes which are the distillation of the five materials, becoming five kings of symbolic images or imagery symbols, thus belonging to the category of image.

In the late Warring States Period, Lu Buwei, 吕不韦, the prime minister of the Qin Kingdom, compiled *Lu's Spring and Autumn Annals*, (lu shi chun qiu, 《吕氏春秋》), which continued to use the thinking way of *The Fundamental Principles* (hong fan, 《洪范》), affirmed that many things in the world can be attributed to the five phases according to their qualities, and related the system of five phases to flavors, sounds or tones, colors, seasons, directions, internal organs, insects and domestic animals, and grains, universalized the attributes of the five phases. So, the concept of five phases in philosophical sense had formed.

The concept of the five phases had been used in medicine as early as the Spring-Autumn and Warring States Period to explain the attributes of internal organs and relationships among them. That is to say, introduction of the five-phase theory of philosophy to Chinese medicine is undoubtedly earlier than *Huang Di's Inner Classic*. A quite systematic five-phase theory has already formed in the *Huangdi's Inner Classic Plain Questions* (huang di nei jing su wen, 《黄帝内经素问》), and all of the fives in the book evolved from the five phases, such as the five zang organs, five flavors, five colors, five qi, five essences, five spirits, five diseases, five excesses, five deficiencies, five methods, five grains, and so and so forth. For example, *The True Words from the Golden Chamber* (jin kui zhen yan lun, 《金匮真言论》) states that "The east and the green color correspond to the liver. The liver opens into the eyes, and the essence is stored in the liver. Illness may manifest on the head. The flavor is sour, the plant is tree/wood, the animal is the chicken, the grain is wheat, the planet is Sui/Jupiter, the number is 8, the smell is foul, the season is spring, which all pertains to the wood in wu xing. And the area affected is the tendons".

(The translation accords with the interpretation and commentaries by Guo Aichun: 26, 1999)[1] That is to say, east in the directions, green in the colors, sour in the flavors, wood in the plants, chicken in the animals, wheat in the grains, Jupiter in the planets, 8 in the numbers, foul in the smells, spring in the seasons, liver in the five zang organs, etc. are all attributed to the wood in the five phases in the way of *qu xiang bi lei* (see table 3).

The engendering and restraining relationship among the five phases also come from direct observation and experiences of the phenomena among the five objects. As regards to the formation of the engendering relationship among the five phases, *The Great Connotations of the Five Phases· On Engendering* (wu xing da yi lun xiang sheng, 《五行大义·论相生》) states that "Wood engenders fire for wood is warm in nature, fire is latent inside it and makes its way out of it and burns; Fire engenders soil for fire can burn wood, resulting in ashes, ashes can be [regarded as] a kind of soil; soil engenders metal for metal is usually found in a mountain which is composed of soil; metal engenders water for the metal can be melted into fluid, [which can be regarded as a kind of water]; water engenders wood for water can nourish wood and make it grow". The restraining relationship among the five phases was established through observing the following natural phenomena among the five objects: water can extinguish fire, fire can melt metal, metal (such as sword and axe) can cut trees (wood), tree (wood) can take its root into soil, and dykes and dams (soil) can prevent flooding (water) from occurring.

In Chinese medicine, the five-phase theory is mainly used to explain the physiological functions, pathological changes of the internal organs and their relationships, formulating therapeutic principles according to the engendering and restraining relationship among the internal organs, thus bearing practical significance in clinical sense.

---

[1] Gou Aichun. Textual Criticism, Annotation and Modern Interpretation of *Huang Di Nei Jing Su Wen*[M]. Tlanjing: Tianjin Science and Technology Press, 1999: 26.

Table 3 Relating the Nature and Man to the Five Phases

	TONES	JUE	ZHI	GONG	SHANG	YU
NATURE	Flavors	Sour	Bitter	Sweet	Acrid	Salty
	Colors	Green	Red	Yellow	White	Black
	Transformations	generate	grow	transform	reap	store
	Climatic factors	Wind	Heat	Dampness	Dryness	Fire
	Directions	East	South	Center	West	North
	Seasons	Spring	Summer	Late Summer	Autumn	Winter
	Five Phases	**Wood**	**Fire**	**Earth**	**Metal**	**Water**
MAN	Zang Organs	Liver	Heart	Spleen	Lung	Kidney
	Fu Organs	Gallbladder	Small Intestine	Stomach	Large Intestine	Bladder
	Sense Organs	Eyes	Tongue	Mouth	Nose	Ears
	Tissues	Tendon	Vessel	Flesh	Skin & Hair	Bone
	Emotions	Anger	Joy	Anxiety	Soorow	Rear
	Sounds	Shouting	Laughing	Singing	Crying	Groaning
	Movements	Grasping	Worrying	Vomiting	Coughing	Trembling

2.4 Jing Luo

Based on some anatomical knowledge on "vessel" and medical practice esp. the application of acupuncture, moxibustion, tuina, and qigong, the concept and theory of *jing luo* was formed by means of metaphor in the thinking way of observing and taking images of the water flow in the rivers on the earth, and analogizing, which is directed by the idea of the heaven and human being uniting and corresponding to each other, as stated in the *Huangdi's Inner Classic·Plain Questions·Discourse on Leaving and Uniting of True Qi and Evil Qi* (huang di nei jing su wen·li he zhen xie lun, 《黄帝内经素问·离合真邪论》) "The sages formulated principles, which must conform to the nature. Therefore, the heaven has 365 degrees and 28 constellations, the earth has 12 jing rivers, and man has 12 jing vessels".

Jing luo functions to carry and move qi and blood in the body. *Guan Zi·Water & Earth* (guan zi·shui di, 《管子·水地》) states that "water is the qi and blood of the earth, running on the earth which is just like qi and blood flowing in the vessels". Judged from the cognizing order, the flow of qi and blood in man is analogized and inferred from the natural phenomena of water flow in the rivers on the earth.

The original meaning of mai (vessel) is blood vessel, as stated in the *Origin of Chinese Characters* (shuo wen jie zi, 《说文解字》) "mai refers to blood vessels running and distributing transversely and obliquely in the body". "Mai 脉" was originally written as "脈" and " ". " ", the same as "派", indicates pronunciation and meaning at the same time; the part of "blood 血"或"meat 肉" ("meat moon 月") indicates that mai (脉 or 脈) functions to carry and move blood in the body. In the medical books unearthed in Mawangdui Han Tomb, most of mai 脉 were written as " ". "水" is the variant form of " ", "目" the variant form of "meat 肉", "皿" the variant form of "blood 血". The structure of the character has clearly illustrated that the ancients analogized or metaphorized water flow with blood flow. It is thus clear that "mai 脉" of the early days referred to blood vessel, so "mai 脉" is also known as "blood vessel 血脉", as stated in *Huangdi's Inner Classic ·Plain Questions ·Discourse on Subtleties and Essentials of Vessels* (huang di nei jing su wen ·mai yao jing wei lun, 《黄帝内经素问·脉要精微论》) "the vessels 脉 are the residence of the blood"(Attention: qi does not appear).

The concepts *"jing"* and *"luo"* appeared later than "mai or vessel". *Jing* and *luo* are further division of "mai or vessel", i.e. *"jing"* vessel and "luo" vessel, which was first recorded in the *Huangdi's Inner Classic·Spiritual Pivot·On Vessels* (huang di nei jing ling shu mai du, 《黄帝内经灵枢·脉度》) "*jing* vessels reside in the interior; their branches running transversely are known as *luo* vessels; the branches of *luo* vessels are known as grandchild vessels".

Huangdi's Inner Classic·Spiritual Pivot·On Viscera (huang di nei jing ling shu ben zang, 《黄帝内经灵枢·本藏》) states that "jing vessels function to move qi and blood, nourish yin and yang, moisten tendons and bones, and lubricate joints". Compared to the statement that "the vessels 脉 are the residence of the blood", quite a lot new contents were supplemented to *jing* vessels, among which the most remarkable point is that the function of moving blood was extended to moving qi and blood.

The characters "经 *jing*" and "络 *luo*" share the same part " ", which is originally used in the textiles. The concept "经脉 *jingmai*" was formed also by means of metaphor in the thinking way of *qu xiang bi lei* or taking images and analogizing. Another part of "经" is " ", indicating both pronunciation and meaning, which is interpreted in *the Origin of Chinese Characters* (shuo wen jie zi, 《说文解字》as "water vessels, following （川）, under the —；—, refers to the earth", that is to say, " " refers to the water vessels under the earth. *Jing* 经 is explained in *the Origin of Chinese Characters* (shuo wen jie zi, 《说文解字》 as "the longitudinal line of the textiles". It can be seen that the reason that "*jing* 经"is used to name the main stems of the vessels has something to do with the origin of the character "*jing* 经", reflecting the similarities between the longitudinal line of the textiles and the running route of the main stems of the vessels.

Another part of "luo 络" is "各", indicating both pronunciation and meaning, which is interpreted in *the Origin of Chinese Characters* (shuo wen jie zi, 《说文解字》 as "divergence of views being different". Therefore, "络" is used to name divergent branches of the vessels.

"经 *jing*" and "络 *luo*" appeared together in the *Han Shu·Yi Wen Zhi* （《汉书·艺文志》）, "medical classics explore the origins of blood vessels, 经络 jingluo, bone marrow, yin-yang, exterior and interior in order to treat various diseases from the root", where seemingly differentiated blood vessels and 经络 *jingluo*.

The extensions from "vessel" to "经络 *jingluo*" and from "blood" to "qi and blood" are also closely related to the application of acupuncture, moxibustion, tuina, qigong, etc, which explore the phenomena of qi and blood flowing in the body, thus enriching the understanding on the "vessels". As regards to the original meaning of "vessel", Xu Shen 许慎 of the Eastern Han Dynasty (25-220A.D.), the author of *the Origin of Chinese Characters* (shuo wen jie zi, 《说文解字》) explained it as "blood vessels running and distributing transversely and obliquely in the body"; Later on, Xu Kai 徐锴 of the Five Dynasties (907-960) supplemented its original meaning in the Annotations of *the Origin of Chinese Characters* (shuo wen jie zi xi zhuan, 《说文解字系传》) as "the qi and blood of the five *zang* organs and six *fu* organs flow and distribute to the limbs", which broadens the contents of the "vessels" from "blood" to "qi and blood", and indicates the links of the "vessels" with the *zang-fu* organs in the interior and with the limbs in the exterior. Obviously, such a change is the result of absorbing Chinese medical theory of that time.

Therefore, I believe that it will take forever to find any three-dimensional structure of *jingluo* through dissecting dead human bodies. Jingluo system or the vessel system is more like a functional concept reflecting a certain image.

2.5 Zang Fu

Zang Fu is a collective term for the internal organs and a pair of specific concepts in Chinese medicine, which was formed by means of metaphor in the way of observing and taking images from the social storing system of the remote antiquity, and analogizing.

2.5.1 Zang

Zang 脏 underwent such an evolution process "臧——藏—臟—脏". Zang 脏 was originally written as"臧" before the Han Dynasty (206B.C.-220A.D.), such as in *Han Shu ·Yi Wen Zhi* (《汉书·艺文志》) where all the characters of "藏" were written as "臧". Later on, "臟" was made to be used as a specific character for man's *zang* organs by adding the meat（肉）moon（月）part to "藏". "脏" is the simplified character of "臟".

As regards to the meaning of "藏", Chinese medical books usually interpret it as follows:"藏 zang4 , 藏 cang2 也", which means "藏 zang4 is used to store". Duan Yucai's Annotations of *The Origin of Chinese Characters* (《说文解字》段玉裁注) states that "凡物善者，必隐于内也", which means "藏" is the place to store valuable and precious things, i.e. "storehouse".

(Note: The number after the pinyin indicates the tone of the pronunciation of the character)

The character "藏" bears two pronunciations, one is cang2, mainly used as a verb, means to hide 隐藏, to collect and store up 收藏, to save and preserve 储藏 or to store 储藏; the other is zang4, originally refers to a place to store valuable and precious things, i.e. "precious deposits 宝藏", "treasure house 宝库", which is the original meaning of "脏 zang" in the compound words "内脏 the internal organs". For example, *Guo Yu · Jin Yu* (《国语•晋语四》) states that "文公之出也，竖头须，守藏者也，不从", in which "头须" refers to a person's name; "守藏者" refers to the specialized person responsible for guarding the treasure house. The quotation means that "*Wen Gong*, king of the Jin Kingdom, went out, but the specialized person responsible for guarding the treasure house named *Tou Xu* did not follow him to go out together". *Lie Zi · Huang Di* (《列子•黄帝》) states that "俄而范氏之藏大火", in which "藏" still refers to a place to store precious things. This quotation means that "Fan's treasure house was set a big fire in a moment". *Records of History · Lao Zi's Biography* (shi ji · lao zi zhuan, 《史记·老子传》) states that Lao Zi was "the official to guard the treasure house of the Zhou Dynasty (C.1100-256 B.C.) 周守藏室之吏也". Its annotation interprets "the official to guard the treasure house" as "the official to guard the treasure house for storing valuable documents and files" ("按藏室吏，乃周藏书室之吏也。"). Such a specialized establishment for storing imperial mandates, files, gold, jades and other precious things had been handed down for later generations. For example, *Zhong Zang Fu* (中藏府), also know as *Zhong Zang* (中藏), was set up in the Han Dynasty (206B.C.-220A.D) with officials known as Ling (令) and Cheng (丞) to be in charge of documents and precious things.

Therefore, we see that the prototype of "脏" ("藏") is a kind of storehouse established by kings of the remote antiquity for storing precious documents, files, imperial mandates, imperial jade seal, and other valuable things. All the things inside the storehouse "藏" are extremely precious or invaluable, which are generally stored inside and not taken out. The five *zang* organs "五脏（藏）" in Chinese medicine function to store the essential qi and not discharge it, which resembles the function of zang "藏", therefore, "藏" is used to name man's five *zang* organs "五脏（藏）" and state their common physiological function by means of metaphor in the thinking way of *qu xiang bi lei*.

2.5.2 Fu

Fu 腑 was originally written as "府" in the ancient times. The part "meat moon 肉月" was supplemented to "府" afterwards to make a specific character "腑" for expressing man's *fu* organs. In the ancient literature, "府" at least bears the following meanings:

① the place to store money, goods, or documents. *Han Fei Zi ·Shi Guo* (《韩非子•十过》) states that "There is neither grains in the granary nor money in the Fu." (仓无积粟，府无储钱。) *Zhan Guo Ce ·Qin Ce Wu* (《战国策•秦策五》) states that "Your Fu stores pearls and precious jades". (君之府藏珍珠宝玉。) *Han Shu ·Jiao Ji Zhi Shang* (《汉书•郊祀志上》) states that "Books on history are stored in the Fu." (史书而藏之府。) *The Origin of Chinese Characters* (shuo wen jie zi,《说文解字》) interprets the original meaning of Fu 府 as the place to store documents. (府，文书藏也。)

② the official being in charge of money, goods, and documents. *Zhou Li ·Tian Guan ·Zai Fu* (《周礼•天官•宰夫》) states that "the fifth is Fu, who has official contract to administer the storehouse". (五曰府，掌官契以治藏。)

③ the place of gathering something. *Zuo Zhuan* (《左传•僖公二十七年》) states that "*The Book of Songs* (shi,《诗》) and the *Book of Documents* (shu,《书》) are the Fu of Yi, the place of gathering meanings". (《诗》、《书》，义之府也。)

④ a general name for feudal official or local authorities. *Zhou Li ·Tian Guan ·Da Zai* (《周礼•天官•大宰》) states that "Eight methods are used to govern the feudal officials", (以八法治官府). The annotation interprets Fu as "the places where all the officials reside". (百官所居曰府。)

⑤ high officials' or noble lords' residences.

Actually, the earliest meaning of fu "府" is a storing system established by kings of the remote antiquity to govern six kinds of money and goods. *Book of Documents* (shang shu ·da yu mo,《尚书•大禹谟》) states that "The earth is even, the heaven is ready-made, and the six Fu and three kinds of things are all in order, which will be relied on by all the later generations to live". (地平天成，六府三事允治，万世永赖。) Kong Yingda's annotation: "Fu is the place to store money".(孔颖达注："府者，藏财之处。") *Yu Pian Guang Part* (《玉篇•广部》): "Fu is the place to store goods". ("府，藏货也。) What kinds of goods were stored in the Fu? Six kinds of money or goods, i.e. water, fire, metal, soil, wood, and grain, were stored in the "Fu", which were often consumed in the daily life and indispensable to ancients' life. The six kinds of money or goods to consume were administered by six officials of six departments respectively, and the institutions where the officials reside are also known as six Fu. （郝宝华：4，2000）

Zhou Li·Qu Li (《周礼·曲礼下》) states that "The son of Heaven's six Fu are set up to administer soil, wood, water, grass, utensils, and goods". (天子之六府，曰：司土、司木、司水、司草、司器、司货。典司六职。) It can be seen that the specific names of the six Fu in the Zhou Dynasty (C.1100-256B.C.) slightly changed, but their functions and official system remained the same.

Six kinds of money or goods were to be constantly consumed, which of course needed corresponding fresh supplies. How to supply them? They should be supplied by collecting and gathering them from the common people. As a matter of fact, "six Fu 六府" were also the tax bureau of the remote antiquity, the officials of the six Fu were a general name of "six tax officials" of the king's official system of that time, as what was recorded in the annotation on six Fu of the *Zhou Li·Qu Li* (《周礼·曲礼下》) that "(six) Fu governs the storing of the tax of six kinds of things". in the remote antiquity. [（六）府，主藏六物之税者。] It is thus clear that the six Fu administered by the six corresponding officials stored six kinds of necessities for everyday life, which were consumed and supplied everyday, so coming in and out were their characteristics. While "藏 Zang" was characterized by only coming in without coming out.

In short, "府 Fu" was a kind of storehouse established by kings of the remote antiquity to hold six necessities for everyday life, known as "six materials"; the institutions were also known as six "Fu", governing collecting or levying tax, therefore, the official names administering the six Fu also had the character "府 Fu". The "六府 six Fu" were characterized by constantly coming in and out of the money or goods, resembling the function of man's "六腑(府) six fu organs" which receive, transform, transport water and grain and discharge the waste out of the body but not to store, therefore, "府 fu" is used to name man's "六腑(府) six fu organs" and state their common physiological function by means of metaphor in the thinking way of *qu xiang bi lei*.

It can be seen that the establishment of "臓 zang" and "府 fu" started in the Xia Dynasty (C.2100-C.1600), was gradually perfected till Shang and Zhou Dynasties (C.1600-256B.C.) according to the record in *the Book of Documents* (shang shu day u mo, 《尚书·大禹谟》). It can be inferred that the origin and formation of the Chinese medical theory were really time-honored.

Huangdi's Inner Classic· Plain Questions• Great Discourse on Images Corresponding to Yin-Yang (huang di nei jing su wen • yin-yang ying xiang da lun, 《黄帝内经素问·阴阳应象大论》) states in the name of Huangdi that "I have heard that in the remote antiquity, the sages talked about and theorized the human body by differentiating zang from fu, understanding the distribution and function of the vessels, giving the names to the acupuncture points ..." (余聞上古聖人，論理人形，列別藏府，端絡經脉，會通六合，各從其經，氣穴所發，各有處名，……。) *Huangdi's Inner Classic· Plain Questions• Further Discourse on the Five Zang Organs* (huang di nei jing su wen • wu zang bie lun, 《黄帝内经素问·五藏別论》) states also in the name of Huangdi that "I have heard from persons educated in medicine the different classifications of the zang and fu organs. Some regard the brain and marrow, the intestines and stomach as zang organs; others regard these organs as fu. People all disagree", (余聞方士或以腦髓爲藏，或以腸胃爲藏，或以爲府，敢問更相反，皆自謂是). The two quotations indicate that the ancient had formulated the meanings of "藏府 zang fu", but developed into different schools as regards to the specific classification or differentiation of them.

All the knowledge related to *zang fu* in Chinese medicine were summarized and systematized as the theory of *zang xiang*, which is usually mistranslated into "visceral manifestation". In actual fact, *xiang* refers to image, which can be easily known by understanding the following four concepts indicating the progressive process of *qu xiang*, i.e. 1) *wu xiang* 物象: the appearance, phenomena the object manifests outside, the existing or being form of the object itself; 2) zhi jue xing xiang or "perceptual image" 知觉形象: the intuition image the subject produces when the *wu xiang* 物象 acts on man's sense organs; 3) biao xiang or "external image" 表象: the internalized *wu xiang* 物象, or the trace of the perceptual image left in man's memory, the image of the object taken, stored and reflected by man's brain after feeling, perceiving the *wu xiang* many times; 4) yi xiang or "imagery image or image in imagination or image" 意象: the result of generalizing and abstracting the image information of the common characters of the objects of the same category, the rational image generalized from the external image, the unity of the external image of the object and the subject's deep understanding of it. Undoubtedly, "象" in "zang xiang 藏象" refers to image, so "zang xiang 藏象" should be "the image of the viscera" or "visceral image" instead of "visceral manifestation".

The theories of qi, yin-yang, the five phases, the vessels (*jing luo*) and visceral image (*zang xiang*), the fundamental theories of Chinese medicine, were all formed by means of metaphors in the thinking way of *qu xiang bi lei*. Therefore, metaphor is a means and process of stating and constructing the theoretical system of Chinese medicine in the thinking way of q*u xiang bi lei*

3. Metaphor: Developing Chinese Medicine in the Thinking Way of *Qu Xiang Bi Lei*

An important aspect of creativity is the ability to create something new by relating it to something already done, known or understood. Clearly metaphors fit in well here because this is also their task. In the field of Chinese medicine, metaphor in the thinking way of *qu xiang bi lei* has been a chief means by which famous physicians of the past generations created new thoughts, and thus developing Chinese medicine in both theoretical and clinical explorations. Here I would like give several famous examples.

3.1 Ti Hu Jie Ga or Carrying a Kettle and Uncovering Its Lid to Treat Dysuria

Zhu Danxi 朱丹溪 was a famous physician and the founder of Yin-Nourishing School of the Jin-Yuan Dynasties (1115-1368). One day, a male patient with dysuria visited him, who was formerly treated by other physicians with diuretics of Chinese medicine which aggravated his condition. Zhu Danxi felt that his right *cun* pulse (indicating the condition of the lungs) was rather wiry and slippery, and then treated the patient with the method of ventilating the lungs, then diuresis was successfully induced, and finally the patient was cured of the disease.

Zhu Danxi pointed out that the disease was caused by accumulation of phlegm in the lungs, and that the lungs are located in the upper *jiao* and the urinary bladder in the lower *jiao*, and that when the upper *jiao* is blocked the lower *jiao* will surely be obstructed, just like a kettle, only after the lid is uncovered, can water be poured out. This therapeutic method is known as *Ti Hu Jie Gai* which literally means "carrying a kettle and uncovering its lid (in order to pour out water)", and actually refers to the method of ventilating the lungs to induce diuresis which is usually used to treat edema, dysuria, or anuria when the diseases do not respond to routine methods.

3.2 Ni Liu Wan Zhou or Saving the Boat in an Adverse Current to Treat Dysentery

Ni Liu Wan Zhou, or saving the boat in an adverse (swift) current, was created by Yu Jiayan 喻嘉言, a famous physician in the early Qing Dynasty (1644-1911), to treat enduring dysentery. He believed that dysentery was caused by external pathogen sinking into the interior, should be treated by lifting the external pathogen out of the exterior from the interior, just like saving a boat in an adverse and swift current to make the boat move upward. He formulated a corresponding prescription named Ginseng Toxin-Vanquishing Powder to treat the disease.

Afterwards, physicians of Chinese medicine usually apply this method and the prescription to treat the dysentery with external pattern accompanied with dampness.

3.3 *Zeng Shui Xing Zhou* or Increasing Water to Move the Boat to Treat Constipation

Zeng Shui Xing Zhou, or Increasing Water to Move the Boat, was created by Wu Jutong 吴鞠通, a distinguished expert of warm diseases of the Qing Dynasty (1644-1911), to treat constipation which is caused by humor insufficiency or heat drying the humor, which is just like the boat running aground for the lack of water. He formulated a corresponding prescription named Humor-Increasing Decoction to treat the disease.

When the river flow cuts off for the lack of water, then boat will surely run aground. When the water is supplied and rises, then the boat will move in it easily. This therapeutic method is just like the above-mentioned phenomena. Therefore, it is quite effective in treating constipation caused by yin deficiency, or heat drying the humor appearing in the warm diseases.

There are many other methods or theories in Chinese medicine which are created by means of metaphors in the thinking way of *qu xiang bi lei*. We can see that the process of constructing and understanding metaphor is a typical example for creativity. The creative nature of metaphor is to find new relationship in two or more existing concepts or phenomena so as to exploit new mental space and advance new theories, thus developing Chinese medicine in both theoretical and clinical explorations.

Conclusion

The theoretical system of Chinese medicine is stated and expressed in natural language with the two major characteristics: being polysemous and ambiguous, which mainly result from metaphors in the thinking way of *qu xiang bi lei*. Compared to phonetic writings, Chinese language (pictographic writing) is more stable and accumulative. In Chinese language, giving the original characters or words new meanings instead of creating new characters or words is the major way to reflect the changes and developments of the world and the means and process of Chinese people cognizing, understanding and stating the world. After tracing back to the original meanings of characters or words, concepts or statements are not difficult to understand in their contexts in a broad sense, which also provide us extensive but close links among different disciplines of Chinese sciences and cultures. Therefore, the statements of Chinese medical theory and modern logic can communicate each other in the deep structure.

The nature of metaphor is to understand, analyze, perceive, and describe one category of things through another. The thinking way of *qu xiang bi lei* is the specific and major thinking way of Chinese sciences and cultures, including Chinese medicine. Metaphor in the think way of *qu xiang bi lei* is a vital means and process of stating, constructing and developing Chinese medicine.

Notes

① *Huang Di's Inner Classic,* Huang Di Nei Jing 《黄帝内经》, comprising *Plain Questions,* Su Wen 《素问》, and *Miraculous Pivot,* Ling Shu 《灵

枢》, is the earliest systematic Chinese medical classic extant in China and has laid the foundation for the theoretical system of Chinese medicine.

② Generally speaking, yin (阴) means the original meaning if the second character in the place names of China is yin (阴). For example, Huayin (华阴) is located at the northern side of the Huashan Mountain; Jianyin (江阴) is located at the southern side of the Yangtze River; yang (阳) means the original meaning if the second character in the place names of China is yang (阳). For example, Hengyang (衡阳) is located at the southern side of the Hengshan Mountain; Luoyang (洛阳) is located at the northern side of the Yangtze River.

③ The medical books unearthed in the *Mawangdui* Han Tomb in December, 1973, Changsha, Hunan Province, include 11 books copied on silk and 4 books written on bamboo slips. The burying time of the tomb is 168 B.C. The books were copied about c. 3 B.C., and were the oldest TCM books in China. Most of the books are stray fragments of text without title. The books are entitled according to their contents: *Prescriptions for 52 Diseases*, *Classic of Moxibustion with 11 Meridians of Hand and Foot*, *Classic of Moxibustion with 11 Yin-Yang Meridians*, *Methods of Pulse-Taking*, *Manifestations of Yin-Yang Pulse Indicating Death* (The above five books comprise one volume of silk book); *Que Gu Shi Qi*《却谷食气》, *Classic of Moxibustion with 11 Yin-Yang Meridians* (B ed.), *Pictures of Taoist Breathing Exercises* (The above three books comprise one volume of silk book); *Methods for Preserving Health*, *Miscellaneous Therapies*, *Books on Obstetrics* (The above three books comprise one volume of silk book); *Ten Questions* (bamboo slips), *Methods of Integrating Yin and Yang* (bamboo slips), *Miscellaneous Contraindications* (wood slips), and *Supreme Way of the Land under Heaven* (bamboo slips). The first five books and related achievements in research were entitled *Prescriptions for 52 Diseases* and published by Cultural Relics Publishing House in 1972.

Pan Guijuan

Discussion of the Basic Categories in the TCM Theoretical System

This paper proposes that the TCM theoretical system is composed of (i) TCM basic theory, (ii) TCM applied theory, and (iii) TCM developed theory which are connected organically. The point proposed is based on the research of the framework structure of the TCM theoretical system, on the analysis of the relationship between the TCM basic theory and clinical practice, and on the thinking of the problem of the history and reality of the TCM development. TCM basic theory is the knowledge system related to basic concepts, basic elements, basic rules, basic principle of TCM theory; TCM applied theory is the knowledge system which TCM basic theory applicates in order to solve the practical problems in the clinical practice; TCM developed theory is the knowledge system which proposes the epistemology, methodology and sense of worth related to the development of the TCM established in TCM basic theory, clinical practice and developmental practice.

Category is the summarization and reflects of the human thinking to the general nature of objective things. Any knowledge system has its own basic category. The establishment of the framework structure of the TCM theoretical system should be carried out and researched deeply based on those three basic categories.

1. TCM basic theory

TCM basic theory is the knowledge system related to basic concepts, basic elements, basic rules, basic principle of TCM theory. TCM basic theory, aimed at exploring and expounding the general nature and rules of the life activity, pathological changes and clinical practice in TCM. TCM basic theory is the basis of the TCM theoretical system. Its developmental level determines the whole level of the TCM theoretical system. TCM basic theory is basic, general and relative stability.

TCM basic theory is composed of the views of nature, life, body, disease, methodology in TCM. The views of nature in TCM are the rational knowledge of TCM to the heaven and the earth, four seasons and the relationship between human and nature. Its specific content category includes five elements and six Qi theory and all kinds of theories related to "correspondence between man and universe" in TCM. The views of life in TCM are the rational knowledge of TCM to the life origin, life process, life material, life activity. Its specific content category includes essence, Qi, spirit theory taking the Qi theory as the core. The views of body in TCM is the rational knowledge of TCM to the body function, body composing, body process of birth, growth, mature, old and death and individual difference. Its specific content category includes visceral picture theory, channel and meridian theory, gift and physical type theory, physique theory and orifice theory. The views of disease in TCM is the rational knowledge of TCM to "health status", "disease status", "changes between health and disease". Its specific content category includes the theory of pathogens, illness occurring, pathogenesis, disease development, recovery. The methodology in TCM is the radical method of TCM in understanding and regulating the life activity, pathological changes of the body. Its specific content category includes the basic rules and principles of the philosophy idea, thinking mode and health preserving, prevention, diagnosis, treatment in TCM.

TCM embodies rich history sedimentary deposits. In fact, TCM basic theory is the knowledge system gradually formed by the practice exploration and theoretical summarization of the physicians of the past dynasties on the basis of the *Internal Classic of the Yellow emperor*. Except the related discussion of the *Internal Classic of the Yellow emperor*, TCM basic theory was recorded by the works of the physicians of the past dynasties for further arrangement and systematical research. Therefore, the research of TCM basic theory should absorb the thinking essence and practice experience in the classical TCM works as more as possible, explore the origin and thinking meaning of the TCM theory, answer the radical problem "What is TCM basic theory"?

The establishment of the TCM basic theory are based on the clinical practice and sublimed in the clinical practice. In the same way, the innovation of TCM basic theory also is based on the summarization of the clinical practice experience and not the simple and abstract theoretical deduction. In another words, TCM theory originated from the clinical practice, detected by the clinical practice, being changed, improved and innovated in the clinical practice. Therefore, the understanding of the TCM basic theory needs the deeply research of the practical basis of the TCM basic theory. If there is no sufficient accumulation of the TCM theory, there would no abstract of the TCM theory.

TCM is the important component of the Chinese splendid traditional culture. Chinese culture permeates into all aspects of the basic theory and clinical practice of TCM. The thinking mode and theoretical meaning of TCM come down in continuous line of the traditional Chinese culture. TCM absorbs rich humanistic and philosophy contents. The understanding of the essence and characteristics of the TCM basic theory and the answering of the question "What is TCM basic theory?" must elaborate the philosophy basis of the TCM basic theory, explore and reveal the internal connection between the TCM basic theory and Chinese ancient philosophy; it must analyze and elaborate the thinking mode and theory meaning of the TCM deeply on the basis of the collation of ancient classic books and theories of those famous physicians. Otherwise, the understanding and application of the TCM basic theory will be very hard.

2. TCM applied theory

TCM applied theory is the knowledge system of the specific application of the TCM basic theory in the clinical practice; TCM applied theory consists of rules, elements, principles and processes that the TCM doctors must obey when they solve the clinical practice problems. TCM applied theory has practical nature, specialization. Furthermore, most of the great innovation in the academic developmental history of TCM belongs to the innovation and breakthrough of the TCM applied theory.

The content category of the TCM applied theory includes the rules, elements and principles of the health preserving in clinic, the rules, elements and principles of the prevention, diagnosis, treatment, recovery in clinic; the specific rules, elements and principles of the prevention, diagnosis, treatment, recovery in specific disease. The main carrier of the TCM applied theory is the academic works of the famous physicians. Rich TCM theory thinking spreads into many consilia and medicine discussion and it is the important origin of the innovation of the TCM applied theory.

TCM basic theory reveals the general nature and common laws of the clinical practice. During the process that the physicians recognize and solve the practical problems by using the TCM basic theory, the academic thinking and clinical diagnosis and treating principles which have their own characteristics were formed. Those organized the rich meaning of the TCM applied theory. From this meaning, the diagnosis and treating thinking and diagnosis and treating principles of the famous physicians is the living soul of the TCM applied theory. The understanding of the diagnosis and treating thinking and academic characteristics of the famous physicians is important for answering the question "How the TCM basic theory guides the clinical practice"?

TCM applied theory is located between the TCM basic theory and the specific clinical practice activity. For this reason, the research of the TCM applied theory can make TCM basic theory and the specific clinical practice activity tie in closely. In fact, TCM applied theory is the specific reflect of the TCM basic theory on the aspects of applied research and theory construction. The contents of the TCM applied theory are the specific clinical practice and special practical problems. The tasks are answering "How the TCM basic theory guides the clinical practice?" The improvement of the TCM diagnosis and treating level would not only depend on the accumulation and the application of the practical experience. It is very important for the analysis and solving the practical question in clinic correctly from the epistemology and methodology of the TCM.

The researchers of the TCM theory should develop the theory research based on the clinical practice and the actual demands, summarize and clarify the knowledge system which can embody the diagnosis and treating thinking of TCM, spread the TCM clinical thinking, be useful to tackle all kinds of practical problems in clinic by the research of the clinical application of the TCM theory. The bridge of the combination of the theory and the practice should be put up between the TCM basic theory and the clinical practice. In TCM, the practice of the health preserving, prevention and treatment for 2000 years proved that TCM would have strong vitality only if being used correctly and innovated continuously in practice.

3. TCM developed theory

The content category of the TCM developed theory embraces the consilia, methodology, values of the TCM history and actual development. TCM developed theory is historical, prospective, macro.

The content category of the TCM developed theory includes the thinking understanding and theory elaboration of the TCM developed history; the theoretical analysis and prove of the actual development, existing problems; the theoretical prospective judgment of the future developed direction, mode, objective, way and method of TCM; the theoretical analysis and evaluation of the inheritance and the innovation of the TCM academy.

The nature, developed law and mode of the TCM theory has the characteristics such as integral, macro, integrate which based on the Chinese systematical thinking and holism, depending on clinical practice and innovated continuously. For the lack of deeply understanding and accurate grasp to this, modern TCM basic theory research tends to "dissimilation". Therefore, how to understand and express the thinking meaning and modern value of TCM? How to judge the history location and radical direction of the TCM academic development correctly? All this should be answered urgently. The situation of the inheritance and development of TCM, the needs of the hygienic and health care, the historical responsibility of revitalizing and disseminating the Chinese national culture demand us answer the important question "Where will the TCM go?" from the theory correctly.

Since the recent years, the disputes about the thinking ways and direction of the TCM development are not only aiming at the mode and method, but the different judgment and choice caused by the different consilia, methodology, values. In the modern 50 years, many treatises were published about the TCM developmental research which were full of penetrating judgment. While, TCM theory research should be developed for solving the questions of consilia, methodology, values that related to the theory development.

The task of the TCM developed theory research is to analyze and express the related developed questions through the theory research, distinguish between right and wrong from the theoretic level, set things right, define the right development direction and insist the right developmental way. In the future, whether TCM can insist the right developmental way or not, it is important for the life and death of TCM, 1.3 billion Chinese people, even for mankind. Therefore, it is very important to research the TCM developed theory. This is also the key to understand the TCM development way.

TCM developed theory research, on one hand, should summarize and clarify the historical process and internal laws of the TCM formation and development, the thinking basis and clinical conditions of the innovation and development of the TCM theory based on the theoretical research of the TCM developed history; on the other hand, we need to emancipate our minds, seek truth from facts, develop the related theoretical research about the developed direction, way, objective and thinking according to the future needs and existing actual questions. In the modern and future days, how does the TCM inherit and develop? Firstly correct developed views and evaluated standard should be set. We should make clear the cause and effect, thinking meaning, modern value, future direction of TCM, prove and clarify the theory from the consilia, methodology, values level.

In brief, the TCM theoretic system is a thinking system that is three-dimentional, open, combines history and actuality, inactivity between theory and practice, a thinking system that changes continuously, unifies the inheritance and innovation. Enriching and improving the framework structure and clarifying the thinking meaning of the TCM theoretical system are complicate and hard. This article is the primary thinking about the situation, all these problems have to be solved in the days ahead.

Ma Xiaotong

TCM Essential Conception and Methods of the Theory

The theoretical system of TCM has been constructed with the View of the Whole Generation as the nature view, Information Ontology and View of Comprehensive Experience as the methodology. The View of the Whole Generation had taken shape in the discussion of Relationship between Doctrine and Substance continually, regarding existence of the world as a process from one to much, and do so to derive the view of life and disease of TCM. The Information Ontology and the View of Comprehensive Experience were coming from exploring of the Relationship between Form and Spirit as well as the Relationship between Human Being and Heaven. The former divided substance into two aspects, information and structure, and prefered to recognize the active law of target by information. The latter combined subject and object and then integrated them in practice. The three theories above have interpreted the source, course and microcosmic mechanism of *integrated conception* (nature view) and *determination of treatment based on differentiation of syndromes* (epistemology) what were understood as the characteristics of TCM, and replenished the ontology as a new category.

Ordinarily, modern scholars summarize the characteristic of TCM as the *integrated conception* and the *determination of treatment based on differentiation of syndromes*. The former could be grasped as a view, and the latter is the description of method. Such a statement has been prevalent several tens of years, and almost has become the common understanding in the main in the clique of TCM. But these two points become harder to remain as the sign of TCM continuously nowadays following that the Western Medicine emphasizes more comprehensive methods in the treatment gradually and the TCM pays more attention to combining syndrome and disease, so we have to explore characteristic of TCM from a deeper aspect, otherwise, it will be impossible to grasp the spirit of TCM exactly and make it puzzled in understanding. The article started from the stand of information which was the basic of TCM understanding, gave a new explanation about the principle of *integrated conception* and *determi-*

nation of treatment based on differentiation of syndromes with the ideas of information as the soul, and formed the concept group consisted of Information Ontology, the View of Whole Generation and the View of Comprehensive Cognition, so that to give a complete and exact explanation to the essential concept and method of TCM theory.

1. The Knowledge Attribute of Information Intrinsic

(1) Relationship between Form and Spirit

The View of Doctrine of Form and Spirit was first put forward by Huan Tan, a philosopher in the Eastern Han Dynasty, and was further developed by Wang Chong. According to the thought of cognizing with form and practicing with spirit of materialism, they criticized the thought of idealism which was derived from View of Communication between Man and Heaven popular widely since the Western Han Dynasty, but they moved towards the extreme superstitious trend of thought with the theory of confucianist divination. Philosophers in the Eastern Han Dynasty put forward the proposition of Relationship between Form and Spirit, and showed their position of materialism, but didn't finish the discussion. Scholars in later ages went on studying the Relationship between Form and Spirit, and build up the two traditions on the idealism attaching importance to spirit and the materialism attaching importance to form generally, although there existed some difference on the way of expression in different ages, and local characteristic in different areas. The two position of thought were embodied not only in the field of sociopolitical life, but also in the field of scientific activities. In the politics, the bureaucratic ruling class regarded the philosophy of idealism attaching importance to spirit as the mainstream, while the people and the part of ruling class without vested interest regarded the philosophy of materialism attaching importance to form as the mainstream. In science, the field of natural and biology including calendar, agriculture and medicine is in favor of the idealism attaching importance to spirit, while the field of physics, chemistry and building technology prefers to the materialism attaching importance to form. The mathematics as the tool of thinking and calculating also has both the form-mathematics preferring to the Spirit Doctrine and the counting-mathematics corresponding to the Form Doctrine.

(2) Tendency of TCM's attaching more importance to spirit than form

TCM was prone to the form basically before it's conformation of theory taken shape, which was manifested typically by *the Description of the Bamboo Slip and Silk Books of the Han Dynasty*. In t*he Classic of 11 Foot Arm Vien as Moxibustion* and *the Classic of 11 Yin-Yang Vien as Moxibustion*, the characteristic of meridian and collateral was the visible pipeline connecting body's top with bottom. But such a characteristic became rather vague which was replaced by some more systematic description on relationship of meridian and collateral in the Classic of Internal Medicine represented the forming of TCM's theory structure, so that there appeared the transforming from the form to the spirit. It should be noted that although Classic of Internal Medicine has inclined towards the spirit totally, there is still rich contents about the form, which just holds the point in values that the form is variable, superficial and shot, while the spirit is confirmative, deep and everlasting. Guiding upon such a view, in addition to the underdevelopment of anatomy knowledge about body's form, theory of TCM followed Classic of Internal Medicine carried on the tradition of attaching more importance to spirit than form, and moved towards the extreme as the mainstream, until there appeared a systemic correcting voice by *the correction of the errors of medical works* written by Wang Qingren in Qing Dynasty.

(3) Intrinsic of TCM is the information medicine

As far as the mainstream, it is easy to find that the 3 classics of *Febrie and Other Diseases, A classic of Acupuncture and Moxibustion* and *Zhou Yi Can Tong Qi* systematized the TCM as a kind of information medicine. The 3 classics were all written in the Eastern Han Dynasty or later and closed to each other, and all derived different mentally information from different angle to make some corresponding adjustment and development according to their own needs. The 3 had their own focal point each, and recreated systematically from 3 typical respects of treatment and healthy as internal medicine, acupuncture and Qigong respectively, and make TCM take a big step forward to the practical orientation on the basis of Classic of Internal Medicine. And the common ground is that the thoughts from these 3 classics went further on spirit compared with the thought of attaching more importance to spirit than form from the Classic of Internal

Medicine, and they 3 had finished TCM's construction of information medicine respectively from the points of internal medicine, acupuncture and Qigong. Different from that the Western Medicine pays more attention to the form and its Structure Medicine intrinsic preferring physics, TCM is prone to spirit and the Information Medicine system preferring to the psychology. Its basic characteristic is the Information Ontology hiding between the lines just contrasted with the Western Medicine's characteristic of the Entity Ontology. It holds the opinion that the information of life is just the reflection of life essence, not to be the superficial phenomenon simply, and we should be able to grasp the law of life activity by collecting information, while it's unnecessary and impossible to restore the information to the structure at the back of information. The View of Information Ontology make clear the basic position of TCM, and could be regarded as the starting point on recognizing the characteristic and revealing the law of TCM.

2. The View of Natural Generation

(1) Relationship between Doctrine and Substance

Relationship between Doctrine and Substance was first mentioned in Yi Jing, which described the two pairs of opposites about the *Deficiency and Excess*. The doctrine has the characteristic of being as a whole, origin and immateriality, so it is a kind of deficiency, and the substance has the characteristic of local, presentation and materiality, so it is a kind of excess. Regarding the Relationship between Doctrine and Substance from the View of Systematics, we could get two results about the relationship of structure and information and that of the whole and the part. It could be found that the structure is always in conformity with the part, and the information is usually in connection with the whole by some extending. In addition, we could also get the internal relationship by compare the Relationship between Doctrine and Substance with the Relationship between Form and Spirit mentioned above. Relationship between Form and Spirit could be looked upon as a mirror image of Relationship between Doctrine and Substance in fact. Only to compare with the Relationship between Doctrine and Substance with general universe meaning, Relationship between Form and Spirit applies more to recognizing of mechanism and the life characteristic of human being.

(2) Principle of Universe Generation

Classic of the Way and Virtue brings the principle of generation to light further, based on the description of Relationship between Doctrine and Substance about both Deficiency and Excess and the Whole and the Part. The classic explanation of this principle is that *the doctrine generates one, one generates two, two generates three, and the three generates the world, the world stays with both of the opposite Yin and Yang at the same time, and get peace and calm when Yin and Yang keeping balance.* Here, Doctrine means the originality and the whole, while the world means the phenomenon and the part. The world we can feel and seize couldn't be evolved from the Doctrine which we can't feel and seize in fact, and such a process of evolving should be called generation, whose concrete expression is that the whole decides the part and would be divided into parts affected by the opposite Yin-Yang acting on each other. And to keep the process ordinarily depends on the balance of Yin-Yang, the two opposite acing force, and there will be some abnormal generation to form a metamorphic product of world with the Yin-Yang balance broken. We might describe all the dynamic process of any system easily by combining the View of Whole from Yi Jing and the View of Generation from Classic of the Way and Virtue, and it could be regarded as a traditional systematic model.

(3) The View of Life and Disease of TCM

Classic of Internal Medicine build up the View of Life and disease of TCM upon the View of Whole from Yi Jing and Classic of the Way and Virtue. What we need to pay special attention to is that the View of Whole exists not only in the Chinese science but also in that of west, but the View of Whole in the west is a kind of View of Construction Whole, which is specious to the View of Generation Whole in Chinese. The originality of View of the Construction Generation is not the Doctrine with the significance of whole, yet it is the element with the local significance known as *the brick of the world*. And there is also evolution mechanism in the system of Western science, but that mainly shows the process of elements construct the whole, but not the process of the whole differentiates into parts as the View of Generation Whole described. So, here appears some interesting difference between TCM and the Western Medicine on the view of life and disease. TCM regards the original state of life has the characteristic of no differentiation and whole, so it is meant to be healthy at the beginning of course, but it's hard to avoid some broken balance of Yin-Yang to take place in the process of growing, and then disease comes and the principle of treatment and prevention is nothing more than adjusting the lost balance of Yin-Yang to reverse, restore or nearly restore body's health before.

3. Methodology of Comprehensive Experience

(1) Relationship between Human Being and Heaven

In the Western Han Period, *the Chun Qiu Fan Lu* written by Dong Zhongshu put forward the View of Communication of Man and Heaven systematically, regarding that the heaven has will and the man have moral conduct, and they both could interact to each other. This is an epistemology system with characteristics of theology. On the one hand, it affirms the principle that heaven could dominate man in theory, and then acquiesces in that man have the right to explain what heaven means in practice on the other hand. It may be called *God and I Integral Whole*, which is also the theory that *man is an integral part of nature*. The View of View of Communication between Man and Heaven enriched Chinese classic system of Systems further objectively, besides its contents of great national unity serving for politics of that time. The aforementioned key elements of systems includes the information and the structure, the whole and the part, the generation and the evolution, while the View of View of Communication between Man and Heaven adds a new element of content and unity. Such a connection is extensive including those of man and nature, man and man, body and mind, and so on. The mechanism of the connection is clear that the spirit of the world, also called information or Qi Ji, realizes the interaction and the system integration in the theory of Yin-Yang and the five elements. Only the spirit could realize such a integration, while the form can not, because that the spirit of the world has the trend of condensing, and the form has only the trend of differentiation.

(2) Principle of determination of treatment based on differentiation of syndromes

The most vivid performance of View of Communication between Man and Heaven in TCM is the *determination of treatment based on differentiation of syndromes* regarded as one of the main characteristics of TCM, and it is the integrated process of the interaction with cognition and intervention. There are 3 kinds of induction and combine in this process. First is the subject-object-in-one between the doctors and the patients. They 2 are independent at the body's structure but connected through the life information. The communication of information makes the merging come true. And the communication of information includes not only the communication of language of significant consciousness but also the instinctive experience of subconscious. The second is the thinking-awareness-in-one of the doctor himself. Facing patients, doctors always adopt the cognitive approach combining thinking and awareness to grasp the essence of disease correctly. The thinking belongs to the method of cutting-in from local following the rule of deduction, and the awareness belongs to the method of cutting-in from the whole following the rule of dialectics. We may get the cognition completely only by combining the both. The third is the cognition-action-in-one of doctors in the specific objectives and condition of circumstance. The cognition guides the action, while the action verifies the cognition, and they both constitute a practice loop. Practice should consist of both the two aspects of cognition and action, which should be the dialectical unity of cognition and action instead of the simple action.

(3) The Two Core Essential of Comprehensive Epistemology

The core of the *determination of treatment based on differentiation of syndromes* is the treatment, in other words to solve the problems. And this is a typical practice process instead of the simple cognitive process. What TCM facing on is the whole dynamic body instead of the local static body component , and therefore it can only grasp the state by feedback and dynamically, and this requires to bring the intervened means into the cognitive process to make it to be a internal links of the cognition. Such a nature, whole and dynamic diagnosis and treating pattern caused to form the corresponding View of Comprehensive Experience with characteristic of comprehensive experience, which was used to carry on the theory explanation to its knowledge system. There are two core elements, one is the value orientation of practice priority, the other is the operating principles of local, and the relationship between the two elements is inseparable. There are two connotes of the practice priority, one is that TCM has the intensive tendency of cognizing objects for solving problem, and how to cognize is not so important if only helpful to solve the problem, and it allowed to choose a variety of cognitive model, not to pursue the formal standard. The second is that the cognition of TCM can't be separated from the participation of practice, and the practice itself is the component part of cognitive process. While the local principle is the emphasizing of current conditions and the environmental factors, TCM advocates that all the way and result of cognition and intervention are connected with given condition and environment, and there is no such a universally applicable golden criterion. These two elements are all formed on the basis of TCM's characteristic of information medicine about nature, whole and dynamic mentioned above. The two elements determine exactly the norm of TCM knowledge system is soft, not rigid. According to the current academic development trend, *the practical philosophy of science* might be considered first to understand TCM as the philosophy guiding principle, and *the complex science* may be chosen as the scientific model to explain the TCM.

References

Wang Bo. General Survey of Yi Jing. Beijing: The Bookshop of China. 2003

Xu Shu, Liu Hao noted and translated. Classic of the Way and Virtue. Hefei: Anhui People Publishing House. 1990

Tianjin Science and Technology Publishing House edited. Classic of Internal Medicine. Pocket Edition of the Four Classics of TCM. Tianjin: Tianjin Science and Technology Publishing House. 1986

Tianjin Science and Technology Publishing House edited. Febrie and Other Diseases. Pocket Edition of the Four Classics of TCM. Tianjin: Tianjin Science and Technology Publishing House. 1986

Lu Zhaolin etc. collated. A classic of Acupuncture and Moxibustion. Shenyang: Liaoning Science and Technology Publishing House. 1997

Chen Quanlin noted and translated. Zhou Yi Can Tong Qi. Beijing: Social Science Publishing House of China. 2004

Philosophy Research of Peking University's philosophy department. History of Chinese Philosophy, Beijing: Publishing House of Beijing University. 2001

Fritz G. Wallner & Lan Fengli

Ontological Ambiguity and Methodological Circularity: QU-XIANG BI-LEI

Qu-xiang Bi-lei is the central method of TCM. Therefore we could say if you read a book on TCM and it doesn't refer to this methodology, and then throw it away because the author does not understand TCM in a deep way.

The paper is composed of 4 chapters: 1) the methodological preface on the differences between Western Science and Chinese science and the framework of Western Science; 2) interpretation of the wonderful concept of *xiang* and its methodological importance; 3) discussion of the phrase and process of *Qu-xiang Bi-lei* and comparison with European ideas; and 4) a conclusion.

The paper is actually an encouragement for the further research. It will be partly very difficult because you must stay on the both sides of the bridge: Chinese Science and European Science.

1. Methodlogical Preface: Differences between Western Science and Chinese Science and the Framework of Western Science

The methodological preface will give you some hints, some advices on which mistakes you should avoid. These mistakes are very common in the books on TCM. The most common mistake is to argue by similarities. From this point it is the wrong way. Probably the most famous example for this methodological mistake is the common and wrong translation of *wu xing* as five elements. You read it in many books and it is wrong and misleading. It encourages people to compare it with the Greek theory of the four elements which is totally wrong. You are on the wrong way, please reverse or stop!

You know that *wu xing* does not refer to the concrete five objects at all, but to five kinds of functional attributes or five changing processes. Then *wu xing* has become five kinds of symbolic images or imagery symbols, thus belonging to the category of *Xiang* or image. As stated in the

Book of Documents ·The Fundamental Principles (shang shu• hong fan, 《尚书•洪范》) "the five phases: the first is water, the second is fire, the third is wood, the fourth is metal, the fifth is soil. Water is moistening and downward flowing. Fire is flaming upward. Wood is bending and straightening. Metal is transforming and changing. Soil, then, is sowing and reaping".

TCM has its own logics. This is the most fascinating point for mankind was able to develop a logic which is totally different from our logics, and to develop an ontology which is totally different from the Western ontology. Therefore what we are doing at this symposium and in our research of the coming 4 years we try to compare them in a deep level. Therefore methodological advices are so important to know how to find the deep level.

The situation is not so bad and nobody should be frustrated now and maybe we need 20 or 100 years to understand this and we are not living anymore. No, it is not so terrible. We have in Philosophy of Science the methodology of strangifcation. Many of you have known it already. We can discuss it later on. This is the main methodology for taking into our Western understanding on the TCM. And we have on the other side examples in the Western culture which show us the boarders of our own culture as Westerners.

To warm up and encourage you now to understand the idea of *xiang* which is very strange first for the Westerners. We refer first to the quantum theory in the Western World. In Quantum theory you find the problem that you cannot say if something is a particle or a wave. You cannot decide the ontological character of objects. Why should we not be brave enough to understand the *xiang* which has also this ontological ambiguity? In difference to this you will see TCM is looking to find out the essence of the objectivity. We must be careful to use these words.

Before we discuss now this typical ontology, the typical methodology of TCM, we must remind you of the ontology and the methodology of the Western Science. You can see that the Western Science is not able at all to make the TCM understandable. You must see the presuppositions of Western Science are totally different from the presuppositions of TCM.

One basic principle of all the Western thinking is the principle of ontology identity. It means what is and what is not. We make this strict decision between what exists and what does not exist. And Western science always asks what is real and what is not real and there is a strict division between them. And Western science makes the division between what is essential and what is existential or between what is important and what is unimportant. Therefore they exclude from the beginning a lot and they don't understand that this exclusion is not necessary. Therefore our scientific description of the world is always based on some arbitrary decisions at the beginning. In difference to this you will see that TCM is looking to find out the essence of phenomena. You must be very careful to use these words because these words are not fitting into the concept of TCM. But we are in the situation like Nils Boer in Quantum theory who says that we must describe the results in our language and know that we are using a language which is not fitting, which is wrong for these results.

Is the Western thinking and science the only approach of doing science? And so what is science? *Science is a procedure that enables you to get a survey, to get an understandable explanation.* – This is a more general definition of science than the traditional one. The traditional definition of science was depending on the traditional European idea about ontology and causality and so on. But in the last 30 years it became clear that these ideas are problematic. Therefore – as we will see during the lecture – this definition covers both the Western science and the traditional Chinese medicine. Because it was clearly nonsense to say Western medicine is *science* and Chinese medicine is *culture* – *both are cultures*. Western medicine is culture in Europe; Chinese medicine is culture of China. To understand this definition of science we have to look to the differences between the Western science and the Chinese science.

We want to refer to three important contemporary philosophers from the field of philosophy of science: Karl Popper, Kurt Gödel and Thomas Kuhn. Every one of them did a lot of reform in the Western science. Unfortunately there is no time to discuss here in detail. We just want to point out that the structure of Western science *is different from* the structure of TCM.

In the Western science it is important to make a *combination of experience and logics*. For Chinese science experiences are also important but in another sense while logic has another structure. There is logic in Chinese science, but you cannot compare these logics to Western logics. To make this argument clearer and more understandable we want to state two examples: Take a look at the kidney deficiencies in TCM. We take three examples to show symptoms that are connected to deficiencies of kidneys: loss of hair, amnesia, soreness of waist. There are *different manifestations at different persons*. After that we want to take a look at the different situation and the different way of Western medicine. As an example we take bacteria infection. Bacteria infection can lead to pneumonia for instance and has the *same manifestation at different persons*.

But here you have to be careful. Here is one crucial point of understanding. The relation between the bacteria in the pneumonia is not the same relation as the relation between kidney deficiencies, loss of hair and so on. In the Western medicine it is thought that this relation is causal, a way of *causal connection*. *You must not take this idea to understand TCM*. The connection between kidney deficiency and loss of hair and so on is *not causal*.

From these examples we can learn that it is not necessary to expect explanation by causality from science. We do not want that you suffer and you ask about the relation of Chinese science. Therefore we give you just a short hint: The relation is a *type of phenomenology*. But anyway, keep in mind again that science can be understood in different ways: by making causal relation and by using with other tools and other ways.

The main problem is: if you really want to do a research on TCM, you have to become aware at first that there are *differences between Western medicine and TCM* that make them *incommensurable*. Let us talk about the incommensurability of Western medicine and TCM: To explain and to show the incommensurability of TCM and Western medicine we want to express the following four essential aspects:

Table 1: Incommensurability of WM and TCM

DIFFERENCES	WM	TCM
1. Methodological	induction and deduction	*Qu Xiang Bi Lei*
2. Ontological	analysis/ synthesis/abstraction	leaves all as it is
3. Experience	reducing the subject	unification of subject and object
4. Theoretical structure	rules and laws	pattern recognition and interpretation

- *Methodology*: If you consider the methodology in the Western medicine, you find the concepts of *induction* and *deduction* – while in TCM not. The most important method of TCM – *Qu Xiang Bi Lei* – is related to phenomena. It is similar to the core of the position of phenomenology: to go back to the things. The named method aims that the things are coming with themselves instead of using abstractions and concepts which are not illustrative. For example when the TCM doctor speaks about a "heat in the liver". This is another world of thinking. Who does not understand this should keep silent because he doesn't understand anything.
- *Ontology*: We want to mention this aspect because for Europeans it is so hard to understand that there is another system which has the claim of truth and a system takes a different way as we do in our thinking. In the Western way of thinking you find ontological analysis/synthesis/abstraction. Instead TCM leaves all as it is.
- *Experience*: It is the Western way of thinking to *reduce the subject* in scientific work. It is the claim to take out your subjectivity from the object. Instead the Chinese way of thinking is based on a *unification of the subject and object*.
- *Theoretical structure*: In Western science we know *rules and laws*. Chinese science works with *pattern recognition and interpretation*. Interpretation is very important. The Chinese characters are some reality for the research. This is a point we have to do a lot of research in the next years.

In Short: you cannot understand a book if you just check the letters. It is the same, if you just look for TCM with the methods of Western medicine. In this case you will not be able to understand this system of medicine. So it is important to *take care of the approach*.

Looking to summarizing this first chapter we would say for provocation: Looking for the essential the Western Science loses the essence. And this is so important for many things. They are looking for some aspects which are on the end for the living system not as fundamental as they believe. This is one reason why in some aspects Chinese medicine is more successful because it is more convincing with the living systems.

2. The Concept of Xiang and its Methodological Importance

2.1 The Concept Xiang

Xiang, you must translate it probably into "image"; but going this to this concept we must be very careful because image has in our thinking another meaning. The original meaning of *Xiang* is elephant, as stated in *The Origin of Chinese Characters* (shuo wen jie zi, 《说文解字》) "xiang, with long nose and teeth, is a big mammal in the Southern *Yue* area". In remote antiquity, the elephant had lived in the Central Plains of China. Later on, the elephant had to migrate south because of the changes in climate, so the people in the Central Plains had few opportunity to see elephant again. Han Fei-Zi (韩非子), a famous philosopher and the representative of the Legalists of the late Warring States Period (475-221B.C.), said in his *Jie Lao Pian* (《解老篇》) that "people seldom see the live elephant, but has gained the skeleton of a dead one, so they can imagine what it is like after investigating the picture or image of its skeleton. Therefore, all in people's imagination is known as 'xiang'". This quotation also reveals the mystery of the origin of the Chinese compound "xiang3 xiang4" (想象, literally "thinking or imagining elephant", means imagination), setting off "xiang 象"'s "imagining" cultural connotations.

We can see that the important result of looking for the concept of image in the TCM-thinking is that in TCM thinking image and imagining are together. They are not separated like in our thinking.

This is the first intellectual exercise you should do this morning: How can you take together image and imagining. Let us go to the Western thinking. What is the background for our division? The background is that in the Western thinking the subject is taken out from nature, in the contraposition to nature and therefore he must make the division what is in my mind real image and what is just imagination. In TCM this division does not exist.

You can see how difficult it has become if we make clear decisions and therefore in classical Chinese thinking a division between what can be seen and what can be only thought does not exist. What can be seen is already real. It is not just a sign of a possible reality. This is very important to understand that phenomena and nooumena are not divided in classical Chinese thinking. What can be seen is not less real. The Western thinking has always this question: What can be seen is real or is not real? And they always take away what just can be seen. You must go behind what you can see. This is a totally different style from that in TCM. In TCM there is nothing behind as the real given in the image.

Here you have the reasons why a chemical analysis of the herbs is totally misleading. If you think you can by chemical analysis make Chinese herbs understandable, then this is totally nonsense. Dr. Kubiena will refer to this point in her lecture.

2.2 The Methodological Importance of Xiang

Some Westerners will think that these are old-fashioned ideas. Then we refer now therefore to the general relativity theory, to the question about the stick being under the speed of light. If the stick is moved into the speed of light, it is reduced in his length. You can show how much reduced by mathematics. And the good question was always: Is it really reduced or is it reduction just a question of measurement and they cannot solve it because it crosses our border. Therefore if somebody says: Oh, *xiang*, old-fashioned, then refers for instance to relativity theory.

If you need some examples, here we refer to the wonderful interpretation of *xiang*. *Xiang,* you can translate it into image but image is not representation. This is the main point. Image is not representation. Here we try to go some steps deeper. And try to give an interpretation of this famous sentence: *tian ren he yi* 天人合一 or the heaven and man uniting and corresponding to each other. The real importance of this thinking is that it is the presupposition of all doing in TCM, of all research. Then every research is going this way that they are looking around in which aspect of nature we have an image which is used for this specific situation. In this case the image is taken as the real.

Now we would like to show you the difference of Chinese ontology and Western ontology. In the Western world, the question for reality and real real one (the increases in reality or intensification of reality) is very important for the Western thinking and science. Therefore in the Western science, there was always a question what remains as a real when we have taken away all the subjectivity. This question makes Chinese thinking nonsense. And this we can see in the concept of *Xiang*. Xiang is not representation of reality, but an offer of reality itself. For the Western thinking, the picture is always like illusion. The pictures cannot replace the thing. This relation between picture and thing is for the Chinese thinking misleading. Friedrich Schiller, one of the great poets and philosophers of Germany, has reflected this Western thinking on picture in his famous poem – "*The Veiled Statue at Sais*" (See the poem at the end of the paper).

3. The Phrase and Process Qu-Xiang-Bi-Lei and a Comparision between Qu-Xiang-Bi- Lei and Euroean Ideas

3.1 The Phrase and Process of Qu-Xiang-Bi-Lei

Our philological work on *qu-xiang bi-lei* shows that *xiang* has a very strong adhesive power, and is a vital part of a series of compounds, including everything from the concrete *xiang* of objects which can be felt and the metaphysical subtle *xiang* which is difficult to grasp, thus possessing perceptual ingredient, rational ingredient, and also indicating relationships.

The following four concepts indicate the progressive process of *qu-xiang* or taking image.

- *Wu xiang* 物象, refers to the appearance, phenomena the object manifests outside, is the existing or being form of the object itself, only after it is internalized as man's conceptual image can it enter the thinking process.
- *Zhi jue xing xiang* 知觉形象, literally means "perceptual image", comes directly from *wu xiang*, referring to the intuition image the subject produces when the *wu xiang* acts on man's sense organs, which can not go into the thinking process for it cannot depart from the direct action of the *wu xiang* on the sense organs. But it is a necessary step in the process of internalization of the *wu xiang*. After the perception caused by the *wu xiang* disappears, there remains more or less trace of the perceptual image or *zhi jue xing xiang* in man's brain, such trace left in man's memory is known as *biao xiang* or external image.
- *Biao xiang* 表象, literally means "external image", is the internalized *wu xiang*, referring to the image of the object taken, stored and reflected by man's brain after feeling, perceiving the *wu xiang* many times.
- *Yi xiang* 意象, literally means "imagery image" or "image in imagination", is usually translated into 'image' and is defined differently by different scholars of the same or different disciplines. It is generally believed that *yi xiang* refers to the result of generalizing and abstracting the image information of the common characters of the objects of the same

category, is the rational image generalized from *biao xiang* or the external image, is the unity of the external image of the object and the subject's deep understanding of it. *Yi xiang* is the cell of the thinking in terms of images, running through the thinking process in terms of images from the beginning to the end.

➢ *Qu-xiang* 取象 or taking image, is based on the direct experiences the ancient obtained from observing the objects, refers to applying concrete images of the objective world and its symbols to express and think in the way of metaphorizing, symbolizing, associating, reasoning from analogy, thus reflecting universal relationships and rules of the things or objects. The prominent characteristics of *qu-xiang* is that the whole thinking process lies in taking *xiang* and observing *xiang*, that is to say, "*xiang*" is the foundation of the thinking, and the thinking movement manifests in the transformation and flow of "*xiang*" and the contradictory movement of "*xiang*" and intuition. *Bi-lei* 比类, or analogizing or reasoning from analogy, is a thinking process, which compares, finds, and catches the similarities between the two different kinds of things, then migrate or move and infer the knowledge of one thing to the other.

The thinking process of *qu-xiang bi-lei* or taking image and reasoning from analogy, the core methodology of TCM, can be summarized into four steps or links as stated in *the Book of Changes*:

➢ Observing objects (*guan wu,* 观物): directly observing the objects;
➢ Taking image (*qu xiang,* 取象): summarizing and refining the image of the object after repeatedly observing and feeling the object (see the four concepts above for details);
➢ Analogizing (*bi lei,* 比类): comparing the things which need to recognize or know with the "image (*xiang,* 象)" just taken;
➢ Understanding the Way or Rule (*ti dao,* 体道): finding the rules through the above comparing and analogizing.

You should know that the theme of Chinese philosophy is to probe into the relationship between the Heaven (nature or universe) and the Man, viewing "the Heaven" as "Man's Heaven", "Man" as "the Heaven's Man", thus forming the idea of *tian ren he yi* or the Heaven and Man uniting and corresponding to each other. *Qu-xiang bi-lei* is also based on the idea of *tian ren he yi*.

3.2 A Comparison Qu-Xiang-Bi-Lei and European Ideas

The difference between representation and reality is an artificial outcome of the Western division between subject and object. If you – like Chinese thinking - do not assume this difference, then in *xiang* are reflected the different possibilities of reality, this is the bases for the importance of metaphor in TCM because the language is poorer than the *xiang*, it can only offer one or two possibilities. The metaphor in this case is the linguistic counterpart of *xiang*.

To make aware how different these ideas are from the Western thinking we show you the contraposition in our thinking, the contraposition in the Greek thinking which is basic for Western science. The contraposition we find in the famous old Philosopher Parmenides because he had this fundamental idea: thinking and existing are identical. What does this mean? It means the existing must follow the thinking. Otherwise it does not exist. This is the basis of our science. What we cannot think does not exist.

Actually we cannot develop this nice way of thinking now for the time is limited. The conference should also have other papers but this is one point for future research - the strangification of *tian ren he yi*. The strangification is a totally different context. What is happening if we are doing the one in the other context? The Parmedian context is discussed everywhere in Western Philosophy. You can find it in Kant, in Hegel and because my lecture is so difficult we give you now a short example from Hegel.

The story is this one: Hegel developed a system of all what is being: a system of the plants, a system of animals, and a system of culture. And then a student had been in South America and came back to the lecture of Prof. Hegel and told him: "I found a plant in South America which is not fitting into your system". And Hegel totally cool said: "The worse for the nature." If the nature does not follow the thinking the nature is only illusion. If something cannot be thought then it does not exist.

There is one Philosopher in Europe who is coming somehow close to the Chinese thinking but he is an outsider at all. He was a genius, he was also mathematician. His name was Leibnitz. In contraposition to the atom theory, the theory that we must go back to the last particles, he thought we can understand the reality only if we think the reality is structured by so called monads which have the ability to reflect all other monads and by this way tried to explain what is world. It is a similar idea to TCM. But again in Europe it has no influence.

The idea is a being is only possible it reflects all other beings and this is a Chinese idea which does not work in Europe. And you can see in the Philosophy after Leibnitz there have been some tries to develop this but they failed because they were looking for objects and not for images. This is another point for research.

If the division between subject and object is assumed, *qu-xiang* or taking image is led by a reason of acting. The intention of acting or the preconditions to act determines the choice of image. Therefore which images are taken is connected with the compositions of the actions. Therefore we must be always aware that a literal understanding of *qu-xiang* in the context of Western thinking (just 'taking images') is always misled, it permits the choice of single subject because the identification of the single subject and 'subject of knowledge' is presupposed. In the Chinese thinking, such a metaphysical construction is not needed because *qu-xiang* gets its meaning and structure by the possibilities of acting.

We must skip over a lot now. We just refer therefore now to the good example to find the 5 phases and Yin-Yang and want to make you aware what is the function of five phases and Yin-Yang. They don't say something about objects. They say: they are a manner of structuring. Because TCM like classical Chinese thinking has instead of structuring by causality structuring by functionality. This is a totally different way. In the Western world you have all the troubles by causality because nobody can see causality. What is causality because nobody can see causality? But we must use it. Otherwise we don't understand the world. But we can also structure by functionality. Then you have no causality and it works.

Therefore the Westerner and also the Western doctor clearly have always the tendency to ask for causes. As long you are asking for causes, you are at the wrong way. We underline this here because you can see how important this methodology is for teaching TCM. This is the one point. Practitioners like Prof. Kubiena internalize the advices of TCM in a way that they may use it in a correct way without studying the methodological aspects but the normal students of TCM is not able to take away the cause of reasoning, the material reasoning and all these things we have learned from the beginning of our life because it is part of our culture.

We do not discuss didactics in this paper but generally an approach which is closer to the Chinese thinking is by the standpoint of practising of acting not by the standpoint of theory because another important difference between the classical Chinese thinking and the Western thinking is that the Westerner takes the activity after the theory. The theory must guide the activity. And this totally different style is also learned at Medical Universities and therefore these Universities are so less open for TCM because they learn this in a totally different style. They learn first theory and follow the theory then they are on the right way. But if you learn TCM you must learn it the other way: Follow the possibilities of actions and build up something.

Therefore the concept of experience for Chinese Medicine is a totally different concept than the concept of experience in the Western Medicine. You cannot compare them directly. A good argument against the use of Western Science for TCM: Experience in the Chinese way is following the possibilities of acting. It is connected with the *tian ren he yi* or the heaven and man uniting and corresponding to each other as presupposition.

4. Conclusion

A direct comparison between Chinese thinking and Western thinking is always misleading in this case the Chinese thinking always loses because what is important for the Chinese thinking has in the Western thinking the fame of the being wrong or at least deficient. Circularity they take in the Western world is logical mistake, in the Chinese thinking it is the bases for revealing the manifold aspects of reality: the reveal of one aspect enriches another aspect as the first one is only understandable for the second one. For the circular reasoning is fundamental.

In the Western thinking ontological ambiguity is only a sign for insufficient or unsatisfactory scientific research. Remark: Compare the discussion between Albert Einstein and followers of quantum theory. (S B) In the Chinese thinking it is – as we have shown- the precondition for the manifoldness of acting.

References

Lan Feng-li. Metaphor, *Qu-xiang Bi-lei* and Chinese Medicine. The Methodology of TCM [C]. Forthcoming.

Wallner, Friedrich. The Comparison between Western Medicine and TCM. Five Lectures on the Foundations of TCM [C]. Forthcoming.

Wallner, Friedrich. The Theoretical Structure and Methodology of TCM. Five Lectures on the Foundations of TCM [C]. Forthcoming.

Xing Yu-Rui. The Theories and Methodology in the *Huang Di's Inner Classic*[M]. Xi'an: Shaanxi Science and Technology Press, 2004.

Appendix: The Veiled Statue at Sais (Friedrich Schiller)

A youth, impelled by a burning thirst for knowledge
To roam to Sais, in fair Egypt's land,
The priesthood's secret learning to explore,
Had passed through many a grade with eager haste,
And still was hurrying on with fond impatience.
Scarce could the Hierophant impose a rein
Upon his headlong efforts. "What avails
A part without the whole?" the youth exclaimed;
"Can there be here a lesser or a greater?
The truth thou speak'st of, like mere earthly dross,
Is't but a sum that can be held by man
In larger or in smaller quantity?
Surely 'tis changeless, indivisible;
Deprive a harmony of but one note,
Deprive the rainbow of one single color,
And all that will remain is naught, so long
As that one color, that one note, is wanting."

While thus they converse held, they chanced to stand
Within the precincts of a lonely temple,
Where a veiled statue of gigantic size
The youth's attention caught. In wonderment
He turned him toward his guide, and asked him, saying,
"What form is that concealed beneath yon veil?"

"Truth!" was the answer. "What!" the young man cried,
"When I am striving after truth alone,
Seekest thou to hide that very truth from me?"

"The Godhead's self alone can answer thee,"
Replied the Hierophant. "'Let no rash mortal
Disturb this veil,' said he, 'till raised by me;
For he who dares with sacrilegious hand
To move the sacred mystic covering,
He'–said the Godhead–" "Well?"–"'will see the truth.'"
"Strangely oracular, indeed! And thou
Hast never ventured, then, to raise the veil?"
"I? Truly not! I never even felt
The least desire."–"Is't possible? If I
Were severed from the truth by nothing else
Than this thin gauze–" "And a divine decree,"
His guide broke in. "Far heavier than thou thinkest
Is this thin gauze, my son. Light to thy hand
It may be–but most weighty to thy conscience."

The youth now sought his home, absorbed in thought;
His burning wish to solve the mystery
Banished all sleep; upon his couch he lay,
Tossing his feverish limbs. When midnight came,
He rose, and toward the temple timidly,
Led by a mighty impulse, bent his way.
The walls he scaled, and soon one active spring
Landed the daring boy beneath the dome.

Behold him now, in utter solitude,
Welcomed by naught save fearful, deathlike silence,–
A silence which the echo of his steps
Alone disturbs, as through the vaults he paces.
Piercing an opening in the cupola,
The moon cast down her pale and silvery beams,
And, awful as a present deity,
Glittering amid the darkness of the pile,

In its long veil concealed, the statue stands.

With hesitating step, he now draws near—
His impious hand would fain remove the veil—
Sudden a burning chill assails his bones
And then an unseen arm repulses him.
"Unhappy one, what wouldst thou do?" Thus cries
A faithful voice within his trembling breast.
"Wouldst thou profanely violate the All-Holy?"
"'Tis true the oracle declared, 'Let none
Venture to raise the veil till raised by me.'
But did the oracle itself not add,
That he who did so would behold the truth?
Whate'er is hid behind, I'll raise the veil."
And then he shouted: "Yes! I will behold it!"
"Behold it!"
Repeats in mocking tone the distant echo.

He speaks, and, with the word, lifts up the veil.
Would you inquire what form there met his eye?
I know not,—but, when day appeared, the priests
Found him extended senseless, pale as death,
Before the pedestal of Isis' statue.
What had been seen and heard by him when there
He never would disclose, but from that hour
His happiness in life had fled forever,
And his deep sorrow soon conducted him
To an untimely grave. "Woe to that man,"
He warning said to every questioner,
"Woe to that man who wins the truth by guilt,
For truth so gained will ne'er reward its owner."

Sophie Chung

Structural Paralellisms in Psychoanalysis and Traditional Chinese Medicine and Their Struggle for Scientific Acknowledgement in the Western World

Initially, one might be confused and tempted to question the topic of this work. It may seem that the intention of describing structural similarities of Psychoanalysis and Traditional Chinese Medicine (TCM) are an unreasonable endeavor in means of philosophy of science given by the different history, origin, cultural background and many other factors that are associated with those two disciplines. However, when taking a closer look, a number of parallelisms in certain aspects become apparent – more than one would probably have expected. The most prominent aspect evolving from a construct of structural similarities is the struggle for scientific acknowledgement among the western scientific world.

Therefore, a short introduction about how science is defined in our western oriented world should be given before going into further discussion about structural characteristics of Psychoanalysis and TCM. Regarding the numbers of books and articles that have been published about the definition of what it takes to be regarded as being scientific, it becomes clear that many more or less brilliant minds throughout history have scrutinized this issue and that the following can be only a very rough overview.

To understand, why Psychoanalysis and TCM are so often misleadingly expelled from being scientific, we need to understand, how science is defined in our western world and that this is not the only scientific system existing at anytime. On the other hand, when understanding western scientific systems – including *hard sciences* like Physics – it might become clear that the many *scientific rules* also apply to disciplines like Psychoanalysis and TCM whereas some don't even for western scientific disciplines like Astronomy.

"Science is what scientists do", which leads to the question: What is a scientist? Generally, a scientist is a person whose intention is to understand nature.

At the very beginning stands the scientific theory. The scientific theory is mostly based on the scientist's experience and believes. The scientific theory proves true through empiricism and when it works out in experiments. As Frank correctly stated, a theory is "scientifically confirmed", if facts coming from the theory can be observed and if there's a great number of observable data coming from the theory. (Frank, 1959)

In fact, the theory is a construct of axioms. Of note, axioms are not defining observable phenomena, but they define relations between abstract concepts like *length* or *point*. The abstract theoretical concept of *length* for example becomes observable when being connected in a process that allows the measurement of the length of a body. "These propositions contain the description of actually observable facts and are formulated partly in the language of our everyday life." (Frank, 1959)

The experiment is the prominent method of western science and thus, the limitations of an experiment results in limitation of scientific insight and *per definitionem* understanding of nature. Conclusions coming from a scientific experiment can only be made based on data that was measured during the experiment. However, an experiment needs to be reproducible and therefore standardization of its components must be possible.

The results gathered by experiments are to be systematically connected within the scientific system, so that based on the existing paradigms and given theories, a logical deductive explanation for occurrences measured during the experiment can be stated.

When for example, a certain protein "X" has been observed to be increased in human beings with ischemic heart disease, the scientist might go back to establish an experiment model in order to find out the causality. He might set up an experiment, where the lack of oxygen in cultured heart cells isolated from rat hearts exhibit an increase of that certain protein "X" (in this case the measured data). Thus, the scientist could come up with the theory: Given, he has proven the direct causality between lack of oxygen and increase of protein "X", he can assume that lack of oxygen is affecting the human heart in a similar way as it does in a rat heart. The increase of protein "X" in the human body is not only a marker for ischemia but the direct consequence of lack of oxygen. What we see here is, that western science is highly deductive and linear in its structure and its conclusions as Hempel wrote in one of his works: "Scientific systematization is ultimately aimed at establishing explanatory and predictive order among the bewildering complex 'data' of our experience, the phenomena that can be directly 'observed' by us." (Hempel, 1958) It helps to generate general concepts and correlations. By looking at the given example, it also becomes very clear how reductive western science is in its characteristics. Not only does the scientist gains his assumptions about the human heart from a rat heart, he goes even further and derives his insight from a few rat heart cells in a Petri dish, isolated from its natural environment (the vital rat body), ignoring the body's environment and its natural influence. Reduction is characterized through eliminating specific quality of an object or observation. (Vuillemin, 1991) It becomes concerning, when scientists think that understanding the model is equal to understanding the nature. This is just not the fact. The model is not a copy of nature, it replaces nature in the experiment. (Wallner, 2002) At this point, a very important question emerges: What if the subject that we want to investigate can't be standardized or what if there's no simplified experimental model just like for the human mind? This is what Psychoanalysis is about. We have to consider the individuality of every human person and unique complexity of interactions that come into play when attempting to understand, explain and predict human behavior. Therefore, Psychoanalysis with its lack of the possibility of standardization of its subjects (human mind) and experimental methods as well as the widely propagated possibility of falsification (Popper, 1935/1994) has been more than once classified to be a non-scientific discipline within Western scientific communities. But the point is, pure reductionist experimental science cannot comprehend the intimate essences of objects. (Sullivan, 1952) The experimental method is without doubt of great advantage when it comes to data control and eliminating variations. (Rahman, 1977) But when it comes to the subjective character of TCM or PA, experimental methods reach their limits. Experiments that take the complexity of human life into consideration are hardly possible to be performed. Even Freud pointed out in saying, "experimentation with the heavenly bodies is after all exceedingly difficult" (Freud, 1933). He argued that acknowledged Western scientific disciplines like Astronomy are not regarded as experimental science themselves. (Rahman, 1977)

Murphy summarized four points that any scientific or philosophic system should include (Murphy, 1960):
1. The scientific system has to define the underlying elements that can be approached through analysis

2. It has to demonstrate the interrelation of the elements
3. It has to offer solutions for problems resulting out of the character after functional integration
4. It must describe the interaction with the environment of the resulting system

When applying those four points onto TCM or Psychoanalysis, it becomes clear, that their structures are not so far away from other western scientific disciplines. A detailed comment on this will be given in the following sections of this paper.

By stepping away from the western oriented scientific understanding, a scientific system should be defined, based on its own paradigms, as a construction of knowledge about nature that is coherent and logical in itself, thus requires its own unique set of methodological understanding and approach for scientific elaboration. Of note, sometimes western scientists tend to forget, that the method of experimental investigation is only one of a great variety of investigational methods that can be applied.

For Freud, the scientific endeavor was to "arrive at a correspondence with reality" (Freud, 1933). It is assumed that Freud was very familiar with the experimental method and the impact of philosophy of science of at that time's *Naturforscher* (Hartmann, 1964) can't be denied. Freud's initial endeavor to find physical correlations for his theory became clear in parts of his work that was dominated by neurophysiology. However, the decisive progress in Psychoanalysis has not set in until Freud let loose from his notion to find physiological substrates and approached wider and maybe more intuitive psychological models. (Frenkel-Brunswik, 1954)

The same mistake can be for example observed in a vast amount of times when scientists are trying to find a biological substrate for *meridians* or *acupuncture points*. This endeavor is not only for the given examples, methodologically incorrect to investigate the structural concepts of TCM and Psychoanalysis but generally spoken for all substructures of those two disciplines. The concept of *meridians* or Freud's concept of the *unconscious* do not require a physical substrate to be directly experienced by the scientist. Therefore it is essential to understand the concepts that make up a theory and accept the co-existence of different scientific systems to be able to investigate in a proper methodological manner.

It becomes even distinctively clearer when moving away from the *unconscious* to the Freudian concept of *instinct* to see that those concepts are not to be directly described through a visible physical or measurable substrate but rather through its capacity of appearances, such as the theory of *psychosexual stages of development* or interrelations and mutual effects onto the human mind and behavior. Also, in TCM, one would be outrightly wrong to measure the temperature in the liver to describe the pathological phenomenon of *heat in the liver*. Moreover, it is more important to outline the effect of *heat in the liver* and the interdependency with other organ systems or levels such as *yin or yang disorders* and effect onto the human body. It is not about a focused linear detection of a substrate but the pattern of interrelation and outcome between the components of a system.

The concept of *instinct* is only valid when set in relationship with displayed behavior and becomes circular with the assumption of an inherent mutual correspondence. This circular pattern is very similar to phenomena described in TCM. A *yin disorder* cannot solely occur by itself nor can it be isolated dealt with. The *yang* component of the body has to be looked at and has to be taken into consideration when it comes to diagnose and treatment. Without *yang*, *yin* would not exist. *Yin* and *yang* of an *indiviuum* are defined throughout their structural interrelation.

As Frenkel-Brunswik pointed out in comparing Psychoanalysis with modern physics (Frenkel-Brunswik, 1954), one of the most obvious characteristic that Psychoanalysis and TCM have in common, is that both disciplines use a fictitious language rather than a natural to describe processes within their systems. Terms and their translations such as *unconsciousness, id, ego, superego, libido* etc. represent constructs in Psychoanalysis while at the same time being used in everyday languages. The term *drive* or *instinctual drive* (*Trieb* in German) is not similar to what it is meant to be in lower animals. (Hartmann, 1964) *Drive* is a concept rather than a term describing a well-defined subject or appearance. The same phenomenon applies to TCM. When describing *heat in the liver* or mentioning the *triple burner warmer (san jiao)*, common words found in everyday speech are put together and used in a totally different context and interrelationships, leading to heavy confusion in understanding and researching the disciplines if not being aware of the concepts and systems behind the terms. As mentioned above, in describing *heat in the liver,* two very common words occur in a context of medicine theory. *Heat* is not meant to be the measurable heat in a meaning of temperature and *liver* is not to be understood as the isolated anatomical organ liver as known in western medicine. Moreover, *heat* in context of TCM is a phenomenon that results out of disharmony in the interrelations of various systems within the body and is less some sort of heat that originates in the liver. Also, when referring to the liver in TCM, the whole organ system of the liver should be considered rather than the liver as a solely organ.

The lack of a phenotypical substrate and measurability for the for example unconscious in Psychoanalysis or a *yang* disorder in TCM makes it hard for western scientists to actually believe in their existence. It is essential to be familiar with the conceptual language before even thinking about performing scientific investigations. One of the reasons for the struggle of western scientists, when it comes to accepting TCM or Psychoanalysis as a scientific system lies in the lack of semantic clarification, the consistent well-defined use of terms. (Murphy, 1960) To a great part, this problem has little to do with the structure of the presented scientific system, but for example rather with the unscientific approach to translate Chinese terms into European languages without being aware of the underlying conceptual language.

Another bewildering aspect that TCM and Psychoanalysis have in common is that the direct observation of the visible doesn't lead to the diagnose of the underlying cause. Excess of *heat* in the body can result in a cold feeling in TCM. Exaggerated friendliness can be rooted in underlying enmity in PA. Psychoanalytic concepts can come up with a considerable distance between overt behavior and its related intrapsychic variables. Also, similar overt behavior can be caused by widely different underlying or even opposing processes as generosity can be rooted in concern for another person or it can be a result out of a defense against less benevolent wishes. (Horwitz, 1963) Thus, the emphasis is not only on mutual structural interrelation as described earlier in this work, but also relation to observation and observer.

The concept of drives in Psychoanalysis makes it possible to take heterogenic appearances of human behavior into consideration and allows the understanding of the dynamics of the mind. Underlying close related mental processes can result in a great variety of external behavior that does not appear to be connected when looking at it from the outside. Similar consideration can be applied to what is meant to be *Qi* in TCM.

Qi is often translated as *energy* but is certainly not equal to the term *energy* in physics. Appearances of *Qi* can also be observed in a great of phenotypical varieties that don't seem to be related to each other at first sight. The concept of *Qi* allows explanation of phenomena through its relation to the observed. A lack of *Qi* can result in lack of motivation, grief or the inability to keep organs in place for example leading to prolapse of the uterus. Quantification of *drive* (Hartmann, 1964) or *Qi* can only go as far as stating a greater or lesser degree but doesn't allow an approach of exact measurement represented in numbers or any other form of categorical quantification.

Hartmann divided psychoanalytic theory into four aspects (Hartmann, 1964): the topographical (*unconscious, preconscious, conscious*), the dynamic, the economic (energic) and the structural aspect. A similar classification can be made for aspects of TCM theory. The topographical aspect is formed by the organs (*heart, small intestine, lung, large intestine, spleen, stomach, kidney, bladder, liver, gall bladder, pericardium, triple burner*), the dynamic aspect is represented by the vital substances (*blood, Qi, Jing, Shen, body fluids)*, the energic could refer to the malignant influences (*wind, heat, cold, humidity, dryness*) and the structural aspect is provided by the system of *channels*. Just like in theory of TCM, the aspects of Psychoanalysis cannot be isolated from each other. For example, without drive there's no relationship between the conscious and unconscious and considering the *Qi* of an organ is essential to understand its nature and functions. In TCM as well as in Psychoanalysis understanding of the function is more important than the physical origin or location causing the phenomena. (Kaptchuck, 1983)

When dealing with human behavior in Psychoanalysis or the human body in TCM, it needs to be seen in relation to all mentioned aspects of each discipline.

What is known as conflict situation in Psychoanalysis can be set in analogy to phenomena of disharmony in TCM. In case of Freudian conflict situation or pattern of disharmony of the body in TCM, there is always one aspect getting out of balance, either being to strong or weak.

The *ego* or *id* as substructures of personality (Hartmann, 1964) are defined through their functions just like *yin* or *yang* organs as substructures of the human body are defined through their functions rather than anatomical topography.

One of the most prominent structural parallelisms between TCM and Psychoanalysis is that in their work, both fields take aspect of interaction with the environment into consideration. As Psychoanalysis has never solely focused on the *inner-psychic* processes, in TCM, the human being is considered as a part of nature and environment in an inherent effective mutual relationship instead of detached from nature.

In a healthy mind, it is a dynamic steady state between *ego, superego, id* and *reality* just like it is in a healthy body, where *Qi* can easily flow an organs are not affected by *malignant influences* in an unbalanced way for example. As soon as this dynamic steady state becomes unbalanced to a certain degree, boundaries for retaining this steady state are crossed. The person's mind is then in a situation of conflict similar to the body that exhibits a certain pattern of disharmony. Different degrees of mental or physical pathologies develop when conflicts or disharmonies occur. One has to figure the human mind in Psychoanalysis and the human body in TCM as a conception out of many substructures, which are in highly mutual dynamic interrelations instead of a firm, static, unmovable construct.

Given the structural peculiarities of Psychoanalysis and TCM, being strongly based on patterns of interaction and interrelation, it is hard to excerpt propositions from the context for investigation, i.e. the analytic situation (Hartmann, 1964) or the interaction with the patient with one exception. That is in the case of philosophy of science when intentionally applying the method of *strangification* (Wallner, 2002) to point out underlying structural or linguistic propositions of a certain theoretical system when taking a statement out of the context of its scientific system and put into a different scientific system. Other than the just mentioned method, where the scientist intentionally explants aspects from their original context, it is hard to investigate those aspects outside their *natural environment*. To a great extend, since interrelating structures play a major role, Psychoanalysis has to be investigated in the analytic situation as well as TCM has to be looked at in relation to the doctor – patient situation. Even if there are similarities in many aspects of the human mind or body, the subtle inimitability of every individual person when being investigated in a – as Horwitz calls it – "unitary functioning organism" (Horwitz, 1963), makes it fairly impossible to devise of matching similar individuals. While western science deals with propositions of the body that can be standardized, such as blood parameters, TCM and Psychoanalysis find themselves working with proposition about the human mind or body which cannot be standardized.

As it is in TCM, the most important reason for the difficulty of investigating Psychoanalysis outside of the analytic situation, is that the Freudian theory is to a major part based on the relationship between observer and observed (Hartmann, 1964). While there is a strict abstract subject – object separation in western science (Wallner, 2006), it is not the fact for Psychoanalysis and TCM. This relation becomes most prominent when it comes to the concept of *transference* and *countertransference*. *Transference* is a concept that Freud introduced in his early years in 1985 in the *Studies on hysteria* (Lear, 2005): "Transference onto the physician takes place through a false connection." What Freud brought into consideration is the possibility of interaction between the analyst and analyzed and that this can be helpful for gaining new insight and treatment. In *transference*, unconscious desires are being re-experienced in a social situation, mostly the analytic situation towards the analyst. (Lear, 2005) The process of transference does not only happen from the one being analyzed to analyst, it can also happen into the contrary direction. Freud termed this phenomenon *countertransference*. This happens through the analysts' unconscious feelings towards the patient. For example, patients might also remind analysts of other people in their life or from their past. Transference and *countertransference* are theories of emotional substitution. (Thurnschwell, 2000) Also, in TCM, the doctor puts himself into a relationship with the patient to understand and solve his problem. Treatment cannot happen without the interrelation between doctor and patient. From this point of view, it is totally understandable that different doctors might treat the patient differently since inter-individual relationships are unique. This also applies to PA, where the patient might develop different feelings towards different analysts and hence displays different patterns of transference, which might effect the analytic situation and treatment.

When observing with Psychoanalysis or TCM, one is confronted with unlinear causalities. Very rarely, it is the fact, that one single particular incidence leads to another, causing some change in behavior or health condition. It is more that one incidence is already influenced by multiple internal and external factors, which further would change the interrelation of certain substructures leading to a composition of phenotypical patterns. It doesn't primarily matter what was the originate cause, leading to the actual state. What really matters is, how the relation of substructures were affected within each other and by the actual state and what can be done, to dissolve the situation of conflict or disharmony. As Kaptchuck pointed out, the question is not: "what X would causes Y?" but "what is the relation between X and y?" (Kaptchuck, 1983)

Freud's theory is very logical in the interrelation of its components and therefore expels itself from being unscientific. Principles of systematization can be found in Freudian theories as in other disciplines. (Hartmann, 1969) Just like in any other science, observations made during psychoanalytic sessions, can be regarded as data that have been collected, interpreted and put into correlation. In doing so, patterns and relationships can be detected and consistency in hypotheses can be assessed to ultimately be able to make predictions based on observed repetitive patterns and their correlation to certain phenomena. (Arlow, 1959) "The complexity and variability of the human organism, plus the uniqueness found in every individual, presents the behavioral scientist with problems which the physical scientist need never consider." (Frank, 1963)

Also, TCM is highly logical in itself. All observable phenomena of the body are put together in a coherent system in all its functions and interrelations. (Kaptchuck, 1983) Highly systemized structures and detailed description about observable phenomena can found throughout medicine theory of TCM. When looking at the *meridian system* the sophisticated structure of a systemical aspect becomes very clear or when reading the very detailed description about all those different characters of *pulse* in *pulse diagnosis,* it becomes apparent that there is still a lot that needs to be comprehended in manners of philosophy of science.

As Peter Dear correctly pointed out „The history of science is full of flips back-and-forth on fundamental questions about the underlying nature of physical phenomena" (Dear, 2006) For sure, the underlying nature of physical phenomena concerning TCM are yet to be methodological carefully introduced to the western scientific world as it has already been done for PA. Similar to what Murphy pointed out (Murphy, 1960), Scientists and anyone who deals with TCM and western medicine has to consider that the two systems are not stating let's say 2 different things, but saying one thing in 2 different languages – and sometimes it just happens to be the same word but in the 2 different languages with 2 different meanings. (Wallner, 2006)

Refernces

Arlow, Jacob A. (1969): *Psychoanalysis as Scientific Method*. Reprinted in The Freudian Paradigm (Rhaman, M.M., ed., 1977, Nelson-Hall Inc., Pubslihers, Chicago) from Psychoanalysis, Scientific Method and Philosophy, New York University Press, New York

Dear, Peter R. (2006): The Intelligibility of Nature: How Science Makes Sence of the World. The University of Chicago Press, Chicago

Frank, P. (1959): *Psychoanalysis and Logical Positivism*. Reprinted in The Freudian Paradigm (Rhaman, M.M., ed., 1977, Nelson-Hall Inc., Pubslihers, Chicago) from Psychoanalysis, Scientific Method and Philosophy, University Press, New York

Frenkel-Brunswik, Else (1945): *Meaning of Psychoanalytic Concepts and Confirmation of Psychoanalytic Theories*. Reprinted in The Freudian Paradigm (Rhaman, M.M., ed., 1977, Nelson-Hall Inc., Pubslihers, Chicago) from Scientific Monthly, 79, 293 – 300

Freud, S. (1933): New Introductory Lectures on Psychoanalysis. Norton, New York

Hartmann, Heinz (1964): *Psychoanalysis as a Scientific Theory*. Reprinted in The Freudian Paradigm (Rhaman, M.M., ed., 1977, Nelson-Hall Inc., Pubslihers, Chicago) from *Essays on Ego in Psychology*, International Universities Press, Inc., Boston

Hempel, Carl G. (1966): *The Theoretician's Dilemma: A Study in the Logic of Theory Construction*. Published in Philosophical Problems of Natural Science, Ed. Shapere, Dudley. The Macmillan Company, New York

Horwitz, L. (1963): *Theory construction and Validation in Psychoanalysis*. Reprinted in The Freudian Paradigm (Rhaman, M.M., ed., 1977, Nelson-Hall Inc., Pubslihers, Chicago) from Theories in Contemporary Psychology. Macmillan Publishing Co., Inc, New York

Kaptchuck, T. J. (1983): *Das grosse Buch der chinesischen Medizin*. Wilhelm Heyne Verlag, Munich

Lear, J. (2005): *Freud*. Routledge, London

Murphy, Gardner (1960): *Psychoanalysis as a Unified Science*. Reprinted in The Freudian Paradigm (Rhaman, M.M., ed., 1977, Nelson-Hall Inc., Pubslihers, Chicago) from *Psychoanalysis and Human Values,* Gune & Stratton, Inc.

Popper, Karl (1935/1994): *Logik der Forschung*. Mohr, Tuebingen
Rahman, M.M. (1977): *The Freudian Paradigm*. Nelson – Hall, Inc., Chicago
Sullivan, S.H. (1952): *An Introduction to the Philosophy of Natural and Mathematical Sciences.* Vantage Press, Inc, New York
Thurnschwell, P. (2005): *Sigmund Freud*. Routledge, London
Vuillemin, Jules (1991): *A Neutral Reduction: Analytical Method and Positivism*, in *The Problem of Reductionism in Science* (ed. E. Agazzi). Kluwer Academic Publishers, Dordrecht
Wallner, F.G. (2002): *Die Verwandlung der Wissenschaft. Vorlesungen zur Jahrtausendwende.* Kovac, Hamburg
Wallner, F.G. (2006): *Traditionelle Chinesische Medizin – eine alternative Denkweise.* Winpferd, Oberstdorf

Culture and Knowledge

Edited by Friedrich G. Wallner

Vol. 1 Friedrich G. Wallner: Structure and Relativity. 2005.

Vol. 2 Kurt Greiner: Therapie der Wissenschaft. Eine Einführung in die Methodik des Konstruktiven Realismus. 2005.

Vol. 3 Daniël Francois Malherbe Strauss: Paradigmen in Mathematik, Physik und Biologie und ihre philosophischen Wurzeln. Ins Deutsche übertragen von Martin J. Jandl. 2005.

Vol. 4 Friedrich G. Wallner: What Practitioners of TCM Should Know. A Philosophical Introduction for Medical Doctors. With a Supplement by *Kelvin Chan*. 2006.

Vol. 5 Kurt Greiner / Friedrich G. Wallner / Martin Gostentschnig (Hrsg.): Verfremdung – Strangification. Multidisziplinäre Beispiele der Anwendung und Fruchtbarkeit einer epistemologischen Methode. 2006.

Vol. 6 Kurt Greiner: Psychoanalytik als Wissenschaft des 21. Jahrhunderts. Ein konstruktivistischer Blick auf Struktur und Reflexionspotential einer polymorphen Kontextualisations-Technik. 2007.

Vol. 7 Kambiz Badie / Maryam Tayefeh Mahmoudi: Strangification: A New Paradigm in Knowledge Processing and Creation. 2007.

Vol. 8 Friedrich G. Wallner: Systemanalyse als Wissenschaftstheorie I: Von der Sprachlichkeit zur Kulturalität. Redigiert von Florian Schmidsberger und Kurt Greiner. 2008.

Vol. 9 Friedrich G. Wallner: Five Lectures on the Foundations of Chinese Medicine. Copyedited by Florian Schmidsberger. 2009.

Vol. 10 Friedrich G. Wallner / Getrude Kubiena / Martin J. Jandel (eds.): Understanding Traditional Chinese Medicine. Consultant: Lena Springer. 2009.

Vol. 11 Fritz G. Wallner / Florian Schmidsberger / Franz Martin Wimmer (eds.): Intercultural Philosophy. New Aspects and Methods. 2010.

Vol. 12 Friedrich G. Wallner: Systemanalyse als Wissenschaftstheorie II: Kulturalismus als Perspektive der Philosophie im 21. Jahrhundert. 2010.

Vol. 13 Friedrich G. Wallner / Fengli Lan / Martin J. Jandl (eds.): The Way of Thinking in Chinese Medicine. Theory, Methodology and structure of Chinese Medicine. 2010.

www.peterlang.de